DIVERTICULITIS COOKBOOK

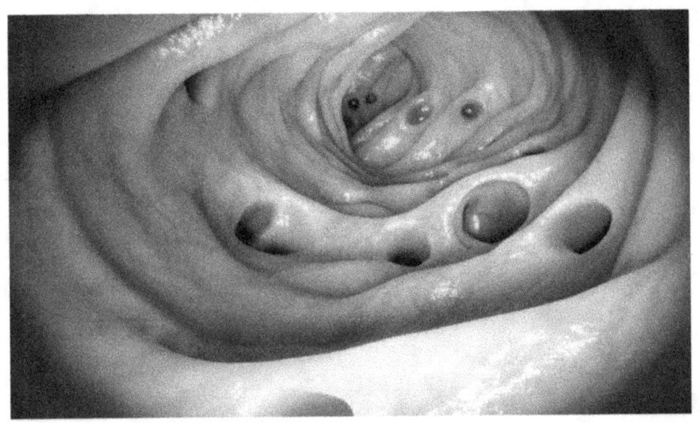

Nourishing Your Gut and Easing Discomfort Through Wholesome Choices

Dr. Jaclyn N. Anderson

Table of Contents

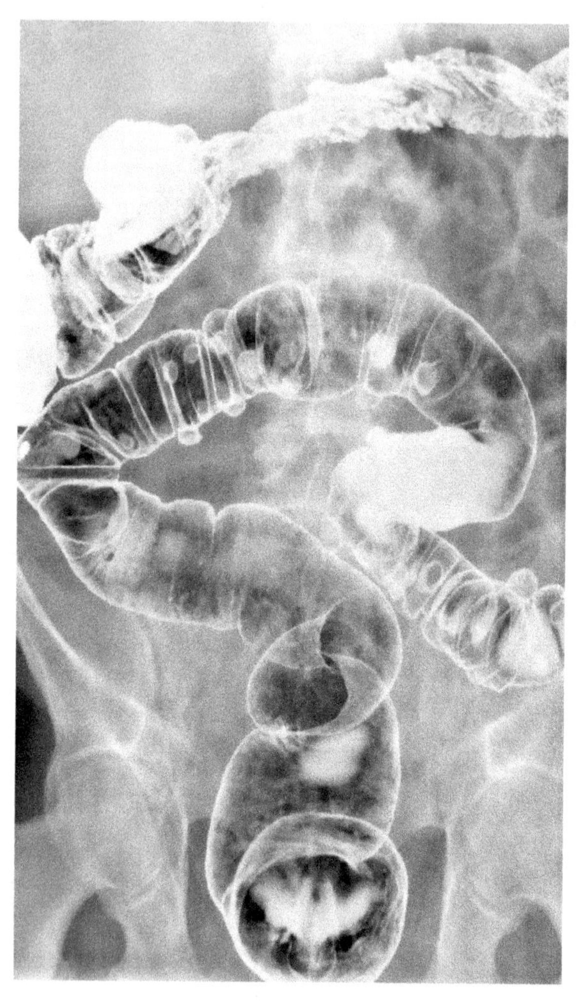

INTRODUCTION

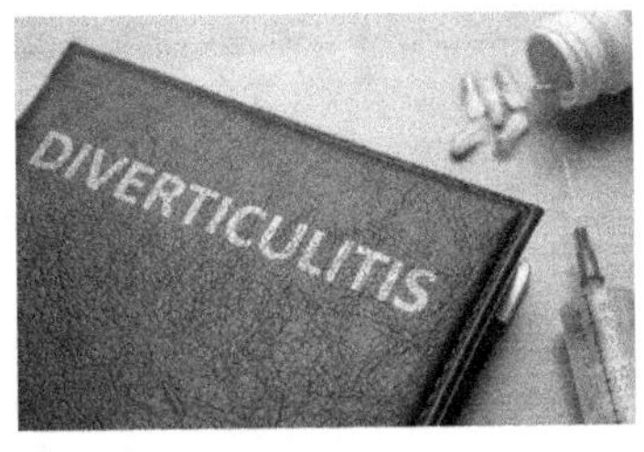 Two years ago, my life took an unexpected turn when I was diagnosed with diverticulitis, a painful digestive condition that left me feeling helpless and anxious about my future. The constant abdominal pain and frequent flare-ups made even the simplest meals a source of dread. However, amidst the uncertainty and discomfort, I discovered a valuable ally in my journey towards recovery: Diverticulitis Cookbook.

The cookbook not only provided me with a collection of delicious, diverticulitis-friendly recipes but also served as a comprehensive guide to managing this condition. It taught me the importance of dietary choices and the impact they could have on my well-being. Armed with knowledge and a stack of nutritious recipes, I embarked on a transformative culinary adventure.

One of my favorite recipes from the cookbook was the "Healing Chicken and Vegetable Soup." It was not only comforting but also easy on my digestive system during flare-ups. The ingredients, carefully selected to soothe inflammation and promote healing, made a noticeable difference in my symptoms. As I incorporated more recipes from the cookbook into my daily meals, I began to experience fewer flare-ups and more stable digestive health.

Moreover, the Diverticulitis Cookbook inspired me to become more creative in the kitchen. I started experimenting with ingredients like psyllium husk, yogurt, and fiber-rich vegetables, which had become staples in my diet. These additions not only improved my gut health but also introduced a variety of flavors and textures to my meals.

As I continued to explore the cookbook's offerings, I discovered a newfound passion for cooking. It was therapeutic and empowering to take control of my diet and health. Mealtime, which had once been a source of anxiety, became an opportunity for nourishment and healing.

Today, I can proudly say that the Diverticulitis Cookbook has played an instrumental role in my recovery journey. With its guidance and delectable recipes, I have regained control over my health and my life. While diverticulitis will always be a part of my story, it no longer defines me. Instead, I embrace each meal as a chance to savor life's flavors and relish in the healing power of food—a story of recovery, resilience, and the culinary joy found within the pages of a cookbook.

How Your Digestive System Works

The digestive system is an amazing and complex network of organs and mechanisms that enables our bodies to break down food into its constituent nutrients, absorb those nutrients, and eliminate waste. This system is essential to preserving our general health and wellbeing. The intriguing process of how your digestive system functions is detailed below.

1. **Mouth:** In the mouth, the digestive process starts. Saliva contains enzymes that begin consuming carbs as you chew

your food. This first stage of digestion helps with mechanical breakdown and also enables the experience of taste and warmth.

2. **Esophagus:** The food passes down the esophagus, a muscular tube, through a series of synchronized contractions known as peristalsis, to reach the stomach after being chewed and swallowed.

3. **Stomach:** The muscular, J-shaped stomach is an organ that completes the digestion process. It secretes gastric secretions containing pepsinogen and hydrochloric acid, which aid in the breakdown of proteins.

4. **Small Intestine:** The majority of digestion and nutrient absorption take place in the small intestine, where the chyme enters. In this stage, the pancreas

secretes enzymes to further digest proteins, carbs, and lipids. Bile, which is secreted by the liver and is kept in the gallbladder, emulsifies lipids to make them simpler to digest. The surface area for absorption in the small intestine is increased by tiny finger-like structures called villi and microvilli.

5. **Nutrient Absorption:** The nutrients obtained from digested food, such as glucose, amino acids, and fatty acids, are absorbed through the small intestine walls and delivered to various regions of the body via the bloodstream.

6. **Large Intestine (Colon):** After nutritional absorption, the large intestine (colon) is where the majority of water, electrolytes, and undigested food fragments are found. These leftovers travel to the large intestine, where water

and electrolytes are reabsorbed and feces are produced. Additionally, the colon is home to trillions of good bacteria that are essential for digestion and overall health.

7. **Rectum and Anus:** Prior to being expelled from the body through the anus, feces are held in the rectum. We have the freedom to decide when to expel trash because this process is controlled voluntarily.

8. **Gastrointestinal Hormones:** During the digestion process, a number of hormones, including gastrin, secretin, and cholecystokinin, are released to govern the passage of food, regulate the secretion of digestive juices, and let us know when we are hungry or full.

9. **Nervous System:** The autonomic nervous system, which coordinates the actions of the digestive organs, is

important for digestion. As the body gets ready for "fight or flight" reactions, the sympathetic division restricts digestion and nutrition absorption while the parasympathetic division encourages these functions.

The Primary Gastrointestinal Diseases

The complex network of organs known as the gastrointestinal (GI) system, sometimes known as the digestive system, is in charge of breaking down food, absorbing nutrients, and excreting waste. This complex system, however, is prone to a number of illnesses and conditions. In this post, we'll look at a few of the most common gastrointestinal conditions that might affect people.

1. **Gastroesophageal Reflux Disease (GERD):** GERD is a chronic condition in which stomach acid frequently rushes back into the esophagus, irritating it and resulting in symptoms like heartburn. In the long run, untreated GERD can cause more serious side effects such as esophageal ulcers or Barrett's esophagus.

2. **Irritable Bowel Syndrome (IBS):** Abdominal pain, bloating, and changes in bowel habits without any obvious anatomical abnormalities are the hallmarks of irritable bowel syndrome (IBS), a functional gastrointestinal illness. Stress, particular foods, or changes in hormones can cause it or make it worse.

3. **Inflammatory Bowel Disease (IBD):** IBD stands for inflammatory bowel disease, which is made up of Crohn's

disease and ulcerative colitis. Abdominal pain, diarrhea, weight loss, and exhaustion are signs of these long-term inflammatory illnesses of the digestive tract.

4. **Celiac Disease:** Gluten, a protein included in wheat, barley, and rye, is a known cause of celiac disease, an autoimmune condition. Gluten consumption in people with celiac disease damages the small intestine's lining, limiting nutrient absorption and resulting in a variety of gastrointestinal and systemic symptoms.

5. **Gallbladder:** The gallbladder is a tiny organ that stores bile produced by the liver. Gallstones are solid particles that form in this organ. When gallstones obstruct bile ducts, severe abdominal pain, nausea, and vomiting can result.

6. **Diverticulitis:** When the small pouches (diverticula) that form in the walls of the colon become inflamed or infected, diverticulitis takes place. Fever, changes in bowel habits, and abdominal pain are all possible symptoms.

7. **Gastroenteritis:** Inflammation of the stomach and intestines brought on by viruses or bacteria is known as gastroenteritis, sometimes known as the stomach flu. It causes symptoms like nausea, vomiting, cramping in the abdomen, and fever.

8. **Peptic Ulcers:** The lining of the stomach, small intestine, or esophagus can become infected with peptic ulcers, which are sores that form. Long-term use of nonsteroidal anti-inflammatory medicines (NSAIDs) or the bacteria Helicobacter pylori can both result in

them. Abdominal discomfort, bloating, and nausea are symptoms.

9. **Hepatitis:** Hepatitis is a liver inflammation that can be brought on by viral infections (such as hepatitis A, B, and C), alcohol consumption, or some drugs. Jaundice, exhaustion, nausea, and stomach pain are some of the symptoms that can occur.

10. **Colorectal cancer:** A malignant development in the colon or rectum is referred to as colorectal cancer. Cancer frequently begins as polyps, which are tiny growths that can turn malignant over time. Effective therapy depends on early discovery through screening.

CHAPTER 1

STAY CURRENT WITH DIVERTICULITIS

What Is Diverticulitis?

Diverticulitis is a medical condition that affects the digestive system, specifically the large intestine or colon. It occurs when small pouches, called diverticula, that can develop in the lining of the colon become inflamed or infected. These pouches are usually formed due to increased pressure on the colon walls, often caused by straining during bowel movements, constipation, or other factors.

Causes And Risk Factors

Diverticula, or small pouches, developing in the colon and then becoming inflamed or infected, are the causes and risk factors of diverticulitis.

The main causes and risk factors are listed below:

1. **Low-Fiber Diet:** Diverticulitis is significantly influenced by a diet that is low in dietary fiber. Stool is made easier to travel through the colon by becoming softer and bulkier thanks to fiber. Lack of fiber can cause diverticula to form, increase intestinal pressure, and constipation.

2. **Aging:** Diverticulitis is more prevalent in senior citizens. The walls of the colon may get weaker with age, making diverticula more likely to occur.

3. **Genetics:** The onset of diverticulitis may have a hereditary component. You could be at a higher risk if the sickness runs in your family.

4. **Lifestyle Decisions:** A number of lifestyle factors, such as the following, can make people more susceptible to diverticulitis:

- **Lack of Exercise:** A sedentary lifestyle can cause constipation and weak colon muscles, which raises the risk of diverticulitis.

- **Obesity:** Overweight or obese individuals have an increased chance of developing diverticulitis.

- **Smoking:** Smoking can erode the colon's protective lining and raise your risk of diverticulitis.

5. **Medications:** Some medicines, especially steroids and nonsteroidal anti-inflammatory drugs (NSAIDs), can raise the risk of diverticulitis. The lining of the colon may become irritated by these drugs.

6. **Previous Digestive Disorders:** Digestive disorders including Crohn's disease and irritable bowel syndrome (IBS) can make you more likely to develop diverticulitis.

7. **Dietary Alternatives:** In addition to low-fiber diets, the following dietary alternatives may aggravate diverticulitis:

- Red meat Consumption: A diet high in red meat has been linked to a higher incidence of diverticulitis.

- Low Fluid Intake: Dehydration can cause constipation, which can raise colon pressure. Constipation can also cause low fluid intake.

Symptoms And Diagnosis

Diverticulitis Symptoms Include:

Diverse symptoms, which can be moderate to severe, might appear in diverticulitis. Typical indications and symptoms include:

1. **Abdominal Pain:** The most typical symptom is localized abdominal pain, which is typically on the lower abdomen's left side. Movement may make the pain worse and it may be severe, cramp-like, or continuous.
2. **Fever:** The diverticula may become inflamed or infected, which can cause a fever, chills, and an overall sense of being unwell.
3. **Change in Bowel Habits:** Diverticulitis has been linked to changes in bowel habits, such as constipation or diarrhea.
4. **Vomiting and Nausea:** Some people with diverticulitis may also suffer

nausea, particularly if the disease is severe.

5. **Bloating and Gas:** Increased stomach bloating and gas might result from modifications in the colon's functionality.

6. **Rectal Bleeding:** Diverticulitis occasionally results in a small amount of rectal bleeding, which is commonly shown as bright red blood in the stool.

Diverticulitis Is Diagnosed By:

Diverticulitis is normally diagnosed using a combination of physical examination, medical history, and diagnostic tests. The typical procedure is as follows:

1. **Medical History:** Your doctor will inquire about the nature and length of your symptoms, as well as any previous

instances of stomach discomfort or digestive problems. A thorough medical history must be given, along with any family history of digestive disorders.

2. **Physical Examination:** During a physical examination, the doctor may check your abdomen for soreness and inflammation-related symptoms. In order to detect a fever, they could also check your vital signs, including temperature.

3. **Blood Tests:** To look for indications of infection (elevated white blood cell count) or inflammation, blood tests like a complete blood count (CBC) may be carried out.

4. **Imaging Tests:**

- **CT Scan:** One of the most popular methods for detecting diverticulitis is a computed tomography (CT) scan. It gives clear pictures of the abdomen and can spot abscesses, inflamed or diseased diverticula, or other problems.

- **Abdominal Ultrasound:** An ultrasound can sometimes be used to check the abdominal region, however it might not be as efficient as a CT scan.

5. **Colonoscopy:** To rule out other conditions or determine the severity of diverticulosis, a colonoscopy may be advised in some circumstances. However, this is more frequently carried out after the acute diverticulitis outbreak has subsided.

Treatment Options

Depending on how severe the problem is, many treatments are available for diverticulitis. Diverticulitis can be treated conservatively in mild cases, but more serious cases may need hospitalization and perhaps surgery. Here are some alternatives for treating diverticulitis:

1. **Dietary Modifications:** Dietary changes are frequently advised for mild instances and during the recovery phase.

- **Clear Liquid Diet:** In the beginning, a clear liquid diet may be advised to give the digestive system a break. This covers clear broth, water, tea, and pulp-free juices.

- **Low-Fiber Diet:** After the acute symptoms subside, a low-fiber diet may be recommended for a while to ease colon stress. White rice, spaghetti, and properly prepared veggies can all fall under this category.

- **Gradual Reintroduction of Fiber-Rich Foods:** Once symptoms subside, patients are often urged to gradually return fiber-rich foods to their diets in order to promote regular bowel movements and prevent further episodes of diverticulitis.

2. **Antibiotics:** Antibiotics are frequently administered to treat infections when there is visible inflammation or indications of an infection. The severity of the infection and the patient's general condition determine the antibiotic to use and the length of the course of treatment.

3. **Pain Relief:** To treat pain and discomfort, doctors may prescribe acetaminophen or nonsteroidal anti-inflammatory medicines (NSAIDs). However, since they can worsen the illness, NSAIDs should be used with caution.

4. **Hospitalization:** Hospitalization may be necessary in severe cases of diverticulitis, particularly if there are side

effects including peritonitis, intestinal blockage, or abscess formation. In the hospital, the patient can get intravenous fluids and antibiotics while being carefully observed.

5. **Abscess Drainage:** If an abscess is present, it may require drainage via a treatment aided by imaging, like a CT scan. This may aid in symptom relief and promote recovery.

6. **Surgery:** When there are difficult or recurrent episodes of diverticulitis or when non-surgical treatments are inadequate, surgery is frequently recommended. Surgical options consist of:

- **Partial Colectomy:** The sigmoid colon is the area of the colon that is removed after a partial colectomy and then reconnected to the healthy parts.

- **Colostomy:** A temporary or permanent colostomy may be required in extreme circumstances. To do this, a hole must be made in the abdominal wall so that feces can flow into a collection bag.

7. **Lifestyle Adjustments:** Following a diverticulitis episode, people are frequently counseled to adopt long-term lifestyle adjustments to avoid further incidents. Among these modifications could be:

- Consuming a diet high in fiber that is enriched with fruits, vegetables, whole grains, and legumes.

- Maintaining hydration by consuming enough water.

- Exercising frequently to encourage regular bowel movements and keep a healthy weight.

- Avoiding smoking and using NSAIDs excessively.

What Can You Do To Avoid Diverticulitis

Diverticulitis can be prevented and your chance of getting it reduced by a number of actions. Promoting colon health and reducing the risk factors for diverticulitis are central to several of these tactics. To prevent diverticulitis, follow these practical tips:

1. **Dietary Fiber:** Eating a diet high in fiber is one of the most crucial preventative measures. Fiber works to soften and bulk up poop, which reduces diverticula formation and makes it simpler to travel through the colon. Eat a diet rich in fruits, vegetables, whole grains, and legumes.

2. **Stay Hydrated:** For optimal digestive health, it's important to consume enough water. Constipation, which can lead to diverticulitis, can be avoided with proper hydration. Aim to consume 64 ounces, or at least 8 glasses, of water each day.

3. **Exercise regularly:** Take part in frequent physical activity. Exercise promotes overall colon health and keeps bowel movements regular. Try to exercise for at least 30 minutes, most days of the week, at a moderate level.

4. **Maintain a Healthy Weight:** Diverticulitis is more likely in those who are obese. This risk can be decreased by achieving and maintaining a healthy weight through a balanced diet and frequent exercise.

5. **Avoid Smoking:** Diverticulitis and other digestive disorders are more likely to

develop in those who smoke. Numerous health advantages, including a decreased risk of diverticulitis, can be obtained by quitting smoking.

6. **Limit Red Meat:** Red meat can be a healthy element of your diet, but too much of it has been linked to a higher risk of diverticulitis. Focus on lean protein sources like poultry, fish, and plant-based proteins, and attempt to keep your intake under control.

7. **Moderate Alcohol Use:** Drinking too much alcohol can irritate the digestive system. Avoid alcohol totally or consume it in moderation.

8. **Control your stress:** Prolonged tension might impair digestion. Deep breathing, meditation, and yoga are all effective ways to reduce stress and support digestive health.

9. **Consider Fiber Supplements:** If it's difficult for you to obtain enough fiber through your diet alone, think about taking fiber supplements. To choose the best supplement for you, talk about this with your doctor.

10. **Regular Check-ups:** Visit your healthcare practitioner for routine examinations and screenings. Talk about your risk factors and any worries you may have about diverticulitis. Any digestive problems can be important to identify and treat early.

11. **Medication Caution:** Use nonsteroidal anti-inflammatory drugs (NSAIDs) and steroids with caution because they can raise your chance of developing diverticulitis. Use these medications as directed by your doctor and talk to them about any possible hazards.

CHAPTER 2

BREAKFAST DELIGHTS

Banana Oatmeal

Ingredients:

- 1 ripe banana
- 1/2 cup old-fashioned rolled oats (not instant)
- 1 cup water or low-fat milk (e.g., almond milk, lactose-free milk)
- 1/2 teaspoon ground cinnamon (optional)
- 1 tablespoon honey or maple syrup (optional, for sweetness)
- A pinch of salt (optional, for flavor)
- Sliced banana, berries, or other soft fruits for garnish (optional)

Instructions:

1. **Prepare the Banana:** Start by peeling the ripe banana and mashing it with a fork until it's smooth and creamy. This will naturally sweeten the oatmeal and provide a creamy texture.

2. **Cook the Oats:** In a saucepan, combine the rolled oats and water or milk. If you're using water, you can add a pinch of salt for flavor. Bring the mixture to a boil over medium heat while stirring occasionally.

3. **Simmer:** Once the mixture comes to a boil, reduce the heat to low and simmer for about 5-7 minutes or until the oats are soft and have absorbed most of the liquid. Stir occasionally to prevent sticking.

4. **Add Banana:** Stir in the mashed banana and ground cinnamon (if using) into the oatmeal. The banana will add natural sweetness and creaminess to the oatmeal.

5. **Sweeten (Optional):** If you prefer a sweeter oatmeal, you can add honey or maple syrup at this stage. Start with 1 tablespoon and adjust to your taste. Stir to incorporate the sweetener.

6. **Serve:** Once the oatmeal is cooked to your desired consistency and the banana is well incorporated, remove it from the heat. Let it cool for a minute or two before serving.

7. **Garnish (Optional):** You can garnish your banana oatmeal with additional slices of banana, berries, or any other soft fruits of your choice for added flavor and texture.

8. **Enjoy:** Serve the banana oatmeal warm and savor its comforting, easy-to-digest goodness.

Sliced Cantaloupe with a hard boiled Eggs

Ingredients:

- 1/2 cantaloupe, peeled, seeds removed, and sliced
- 1 hard-boiled egg
- Salt and pepper to taste (optional)

Instructions:

1. **Prepare the Cantaloupe:**

- Cut the cantaloupe in half and scoop out the seeds with a spoon.
- Slice the peeled cantaloupe into thin, bite-sized pieces. You can cut it into wedges or cubes, depending on your preference.

2. **Hard-Boil the Egg:**

- Place an egg in a small saucepan and cover it with cold water.

- Place the saucepan on the stove over medium-high heat and bring the water to a boil.

- Once the water is boiling, reduce the heat to low, cover the saucepan with a lid, and let it simmer for about 9-12 minutes.

- After the cooking time, remove the saucepan from the heat and immediately transfer the egg to a bowl of ice water to cool.

- Once the egg is cool, peel it, and cut it into slices.

3. **Assemble the Dish:**

- Arrange the sliced cantaloupe on a plate or in a bowl.

- Place the sliced hard-boiled egg on top of the cantaloupe slices.

4. **Season (Optional):** If desired, you can season the dish with a pinch of salt and pepper to taste. Keep in mind that some individuals with diverticulitis may prefer to omit these seasonings to avoid any potential irritation.

5. **Serve:** Your sliced cantaloupe with a hard-boiled egg is ready to be served. Enjoy this simple and soothing meal.

Greek Yogurt Parfait

Ingredients:

- 1 cup of plain Greek yogurt (low-fat or full-fat, depending on your preference)
- 1/2 cup of soft, ripe fruit (e.g., mashed banana, cooked and mashed apples, or applesauce)
- 1 tablespoon of honey (optional, for sweetness)

- 2 tablespoons of finely chopped nuts (e.g., almonds or walnuts) (optional, for added texture and healthy fats)
- A pinch of ground cinnamon (optional, for flavor)
- A few fresh berries or other soft fruits for garnish (optional)

Instructions:

1. **Prepare the Fruit:**

- Choose a soft, ripe fruit of your choice. You can use mashed banana, cooked and mashed apples, or unsweetened applesauce. These options are gentle on the digestive system.
- If using apples, peel, core, and cook them until soft, then mash them into applesauce. Let them cool before using in the parfait.

2. **Layer the Parfait:**

- Start by adding a layer of Greek yogurt to a glass or bowl, creating the base of your parfait.

- Next, spoon a layer of the mashed or soft fruit on top of the yogurt.

3. **Add Honey (Optional):** If you prefer a sweeter parfait, you can drizzle honey over the fruit layer. Start with 1 tablespoon and adjust to your taste.

4. **Optional Nut Layer:** If you'd like to add some texture and healthy fats, sprinkle finely chopped nuts (e.g., almonds or walnuts) on top of the fruit layer.

5. **Sprinkle Cinnamon (Optional):** For additional flavor, you can add a pinch of ground cinnamon over the nuts or fruit.

6. **Repeat Layers (Optional):** If your glass or bowl allows, you can repeat the layering process with another layer of yogurt, fruit, honey, nuts, and cinnamon.

7. **Garnish (Optional):** Finish by garnishing the parfait with a few fresh berries or additional soft fruits for added visual appeal and flavor.

8. **Serve:** Your Greek yogurt parfait is ready to be enjoyed. Serve it immediately or refrigerate it briefly if you prefer it chilled.

Ginger, Mushroom and Cauliflower Broth

Ingredients:

- 1 tablespoon olive oil
- 1 small onion, finely chopped
- 2 cloves garlic, minced
- 1-inch piece of fresh ginger, peeled and minced (or more to taste)
- 8 oz (about 2 cups) white mushrooms, sliced
- 2 cups cauliflower florets

- 4 cups low-sodium vegetable broth
- Salt and pepper to taste
- Fresh parsley or chives for garnish (optional)

Instructions:

1. **Prepare the Vegetables:**
- Heat the olive oil in a large soup pot or saucepan over medium heat.
- Add the chopped onion and sauté for 2-3 minutes until it becomes translucent.
2. **Add Aromatics:** Stir in the minced garlic and fresh ginger. Sauté for another 1-2 minutes until fragrant.
3. **Cook Mushrooms and Cauliflower:** Add the sliced mushrooms and cauliflower florets to the pot. Continue to cook for about 5-7 minutes, stirring

occasionally, until the mushrooms have softened and the cauliflower begins to turn golden.

4. **Pour in Vegetable Broth:** Pour the low-sodium vegetable broth into the pot, covering the sautéed vegetables. Bring the mixture to a gentle boil.

5. **Simmer:** Reduce the heat to low, cover the pot with a lid, and let the broth simmer for about 20-25 minutes, or until the cauliflower is tender and can be easily pierced with a fork.

6. **Blend the Soup:** Carefully use an immersion blender to puree the soup until smooth. Alternatively, you can transfer the mixture in batches to a blender and blend until smooth. Be cautious when blending hot liquids to avoid splattering.

7. **Season and Garnish:**

- Season the soup with salt and pepper to taste. Adjust the seasoning according to your preference.

- If desired, garnish the soup with fresh parsley or chives for added flavor and presentation.

8. **Serve:** Your ginger, mushroom, and cauliflower broth is ready to be served. Ladle it into bowls and enjoy while it's warm and comforting.

Applesauce Pancakes

Ingredients:

- 1 cup all-purpose flour
- 1 teaspoon baking powder
- 1/2 teaspoon baking soda
- 1/4 teaspoon salt (optional)
- 1/2 teaspoon ground cinnamon (optional)
- 1/2 cup unsweetened applesauce

- 1/2 cup low-fat or lactose-free milk (or a milk substitute like almond milk)
- 1 large egg
- 2 tablespoons honey or maple syrup (optional, for sweetness)
- 1 teaspoon vanilla extract (optional)
- Cooking oil or butter for the griddle or skillet

Instructions:

1. **Combine Dry Ingredients:** In a mixing bowl, whisk together the all-purpose flour, baking powder, baking soda, salt (if using), and ground cinnamon (if using). The cinnamon adds a pleasant flavor, but it's optional if you prefer a milder taste.

2. **Mix Wet Ingredients:** In another bowl, combine the unsweetened applesauce, low-fat milk, egg, honey or maple syrup

(if using), and vanilla extract (if using). Mix until the wet ingredients are well incorporated.

3. **Combine Dry and Wet Ingredients:** Pour the wet ingredients into the dry ingredients. Stir until just combined. Be careful not to overmix; it's okay if there are a few lumps in the batter.

4. **Preheat the Griddle or Skillet:** Preheat a griddle or non-stick skillet over medium-high heat. Lightly grease it with cooking oil or butter.

5. **Cook the Pancakes:** Pour about 1/4 cup of the pancake batter onto the preheated griddle for each pancake. Use the back of a spoon to spread the batter slightly, forming a round shape.

6. **Cook Until Bubbles Form:** Cook the pancakes until you see bubbles forming on the surface, usually after 2-3 minutes.

7. **Flip and Continue Cooking:** Carefully flip the pancakes with a spatula and cook for an additional 1-2 minutes on the other side, or until they are golden brown and cooked through.

8. **Serve Warm:** Transfer the pancakes to a plate, and keep them warm. You can serve them with additional applesauce, fresh fruit, or a drizzle of honey or maple syrup if desired.

9. **Enjoy:** Your applesauce pancakes are ready to be enjoyed. They're soft, moist, and suitable for individuals with diverticulitis.

Cottage Cheese and Fruit

1. Cottage Cheese and Mashed Banana:

Ingredients:

- 1/2 cup of low-fat or lactose-free cottage cheese
- 1 ripe banana, mashed
- 1-2 tablespoons of honey or maple syrup (optional, for sweetness)
- A pinch of ground cinnamon (optional, for flavor)
- Chopped nuts (e.g., almonds or walnuts) for added texture (optional)

Instructions:

1. In a bowl, combine the low-fat or lactose-free cottage cheese and the mashed ripe banana. The banana adds natural sweetness and creaminess to the cottage cheese.

2. If you prefer a sweeter dish, you can drizzle honey or maple syrup over the mixture. Start with 1-2 tablespoons and adjust to your taste.

3. Optionally, sprinkle a pinch of ground cinnamon over the top for added flavor.

4. If you like some texture in your dish, consider adding chopped nuts (e.g., almonds or walnuts) for a pleasant crunch.

5. Mix all the ingredients well until they are evenly combined.

6. Serve your cottage cheese and mashed banana mixture immediately. It's a delicious and easy-to-digest combination that can be enjoyed as a snack or a light meal.

2. Cottage Cheese with Soft Berries:

Ingredients:

- 1/2 cup of low-fat or lactose-free cottage cheese
- 1/2 cup of soft berries (e.g., blueberries, raspberries, or strawberries)
- 1-2 tablespoons of honey or maple syrup (optional, for sweetness)
- A few fresh mint leaves for garnish (optional)

Instructions:

1. In a bowl, place the low-fat or lactose-free cottage cheese.
2. Add your choice of soft berries (e.g., blueberries, raspberries, or strawberries) to the cottage cheese. These fruits are generally gentle on the digestive system.

3. If you prefer a sweeter flavor, drizzle honey or maple syrup over the cottage cheese and berries. Adjust the sweetness to your liking.

4. For a fresh touch, garnish the dish with a few fresh mint leaves.

5. Gently mix the ingredients to combine them while being careful not to crush the berries completely.

6. Serve your cottage cheese with soft berries immediately. It's a delightful and refreshing option that's perfect for a light meal or a healthy snack.

Cream of Rice

Ingredients:

- 1/2 cup rice cereal (plain, unsweetened)
- 2 cups water or low-fat milk (or a milk substitute like almond milk)
- A pinch of salt (optional, for flavor)

- Honey or maple syrup (optional, for sweetness)
- Cinnamon or nutmeg (optional, for flavor)

Instructions:

1. **Combine Rice Cereal and Liquid:** In a saucepan, combine the rice cereal and water or low-fat milk (or milk substitute). If you prefer a creamier consistency, you can use milk instead of water.

2. **Add Salt (Optional):** If desired, you can add a pinch of salt to the mixture for added flavor. However, some individuals with diverticulitis may prefer to omit salt to reduce irritation.

3. **Cook Over Medium Heat:** Place the saucepan over medium heat and stir the

mixture continuously. Bring it to a gentle boil while stirring.

4. **Reduce Heat and Simmer:** Once it starts boiling, reduce the heat to low and let the mixture simmer. Continue to stir occasionally to prevent sticking and ensure even cooking.

5. **Cook Until Thickened:** Cook the rice cereal for about 5-7 minutes or until it reaches your desired thickness. You can adjust the thickness by adding more liquid if needed.

6. **Sweeten and Flavor (Optional):** If you prefer a sweeter flavor, you can add honey or maple syrup to taste. Start with 1-2 tablespoons and adjust to your liking.

7. **Add Spices (Optional):** For extra flavor, you can sprinkle a pinch of cinnamon or nutmeg over the cream of rice just before serving.

8. **Serve Warm:** Your cream of rice is now ready to be served. It should have a creamy and smooth consistency.

9. Enjoy: Serve the cream of rice warm, and you can garnish it with additional honey or a sprinkle of cinnamon if desired.

Smoothie Bowl

Ingredients:

For the Smoothie Base:

- 1/2 cup plain Greek yogurt (low-fat or lactose-free, if preferred)
- 1 ripe banana, peeled and sliced
- 1/2 cup soft fruit (e.g., cooked and mashed apple, mashed pear, or berries)
- 1/2 cup low-fat or lactose-free milk (or a milk substitute like almond milk)
- 1-2 tablespoons honey or maple syrup (optional, for sweetness)

- A handful of ice cubes (optional, for thickness)

For Toppings:
- Soft fruits (e.g., berries, sliced banana)
- Chopped nuts (e.g., almonds or walnuts)
- Ground flaxseed or chia seeds (optional, for added fiber)
- Unsweetened shredded coconut (optional)
- Fresh mint leaves (optional, for garnish)

Instructions:

1. **Prepare the Smoothie Base:**
- In a blender, combine the plain Greek yogurt, sliced banana, soft fruit (e.g., mashed apple or pear), low-fat or lactose-free milk (or milk substitute), and honey or maple syrup (if using).

- Optionally, add a handful of ice cubes to the blender to thicken the smoothie.

2. **Blend Until Smooth:** Blend all the ingredients until you achieve a smooth and creamy consistency. Adjust the sweetness with honey or maple syrup to your taste.

3. **Pour Into A Bowl:** Pour the smoothie into a bowl.

4. **Add Toppings:** Decorate your smoothie bowl with toppings of your choice. Soft fruits like berries or sliced banana work well. You can also add chopped nuts for texture, ground flaxseed or chia seeds for added fiber, and a sprinkle of unsweetened shredded coconut for flavor.

5. **Garnish (Optional):** For a fresh touch, garnish the smoothie bowl with a few fresh mint leaves.

6. **Serve:** Your smoothie bowl is ready to be served. Enjoy it while it's fresh and delicious.

Chia Seed Pudding

Ingredients:

- 2 tablespoons chia seeds
- 1/2 cup low-fat or lactose-free milk (or a milk substitute like almond milk)
- 1-2 tablespoons honey or maple syrup (optional, for sweetness)
- 1/2 teaspoon vanilla extract (optional, for flavor)
- Soft fruits (e.g., mashed banana, cooked and mashed apples, or berries) for added flavor and texture (optional)
- Chopped nuts (e.g., almonds or walnuts) for added texture (optional)
- A pinch of ground cinnamon (optional, for flavor)

Instructions:

1. **Combine Chia Seeds and Liquid:** In a bowl or a jar, combine the chia seeds and low-fat or lactose-free milk (or milk substitute). If you prefer a creamier consistency, you can use milk instead of water.

2. **Add Sweetener (Optional):** If desired, add honey or maple syrup to the mixture for added sweetness. Start with 1-2 tablespoons and adjust to your taste.

3. **Flavor with Vanilla (Optional):** To enhance the flavor, you can add vanilla extract to the mixture. Mix it in well.

4. **Soak Chia Seeds:**

- Stir the ingredients together until the chia seeds are evenly distributed in the liquid. Make sure there are no clumps of seeds.

- Let the mixture sit for a few minutes to allow the chia seeds to absorb the liquid. Stir again to prevent clumping.

5. **Add Soft Fruits (Optional):** To enhance the flavor and texture, consider adding soft fruits like mashed banana, cooked and mashed apples, or berries to the mixture. These fruits are generally gentle on the digestive system.

6. **Chill and Thicken:** Cover the bowl or jar and refrigerate the mixture for at least 2-3 hours, or ideally overnight. This allows the chia seeds to absorb more liquid and create a pudding-like texture.

7. **Serve and Customize:**

- When ready to serve, give the chia pudding a good stir to redistribute the seeds evenly.

- You can garnish your chia seed pudding with chopped nuts (e.g., almonds or walnuts) for added texture and flavor. A pinch of ground cinnamon can also be sprinkled on top for extra flavor.

8. **Enjoy:** Your chia seed pudding is ready to be enjoyed. It's a creamy and nutritious treat suitable for individuals with diverticulitis.

Indian Inspired Vegetable Stock

Ingredients:

- 8 cups water
- 2 large carrots, chopped
- 2 celery stalks, chopped
- 1 large onion, chopped
- 1 medium potato, chopped
- 1 large tomato, chopped
- 2 cloves garlic, minced
- 1-inch piece of ginger, sliced
- 1/2 teaspoon ground cumin
- 1/2 teaspoon ground coriander

- 1/2 teaspoon ground turmeric

- 1/2 teaspoon ground cinnamon

- 1/4 teaspoon ground cardamom

- 1/4 teaspoon ground cloves

- 1/4 teaspoon ground black pepper

- 1 bay leaf

- 1-2 dried red chilies (adjust to your spice preference, or omit if sensitive)

- A handful of fresh cilantro or parsley stems

- Salt to taste

- 1-2 tablespoons olive oil or vegetable oil

Instructions:

1. **Sauté the Aromatics:** In a large pot or Dutch oven, heat the olive oil over medium heat. Add the minced garlic and sliced ginger. Sauté for a minute or until fragrant.

2. **Add Spices:** Add the ground cumin, ground coriander, ground turmeric, ground cinnamon, ground cardamom, ground cloves, ground black pepper, and dried red chilies (if using). Stir and cook for another minute until the spices release their aroma.

3. **Add Chopped Vegetables:** Add the chopped carrots, celery, onion, potato, and tomato to the pot. Stir well to coat the vegetables with the aromatic spices.

4. **Pour in Water:** Pour in 8 cups of water, ensuring the vegetables are submerged.

5. **Add Bay Leaf and Fresh Herbs:** Toss in the bay leaf and a handful of fresh cilantro or parsley stems. These herbs will impart a fresh flavor to the stock. Reserve the leaves for garnish.

6. **Simmer:** Bring the mixture to a boil, then reduce the heat to low. Cover the

pot and let the stock simmer for about 30-40 minutes. The vegetables should become tender, and the flavors should meld together.

7. **Strain:** Once the stock is ready, strain it through a fine-mesh sieve or cheesecloth into another pot or container. Discard the solids or save them for another use.

8. **Season with Salt:** Taste the vegetable stock and season it with salt as needed. Add a little at a time, tasting between additions to achieve your desired saltiness.

9. **Cool and Store:** Allow the stock to cool to room temperature before storing it in airtight containers. You can refrigerate it for up to 3-4 days or freeze it for longer storage.

10. **Use in Recipes:** Use your homemade Indian-inspired vegetable stock as a base

for soups, stews, curries, or other dishes that call for stock or broth. It will add rich flavor with a touch of Indian spice.

Scrambled Tofu

Ingredients:

- 1 block of extra-firm tofu (14-16 ounces), drained and pressed
- 2 tablespoons olive oil or vegetable oil
- 1/2 onion, finely chopped
- 1/2 bell pepper, finely chopped (choose a color you prefer)
- 1/2 teaspoon ground turmeric (for color and flavor)
- Salt and pepper to taste
- Chopped fresh parsley or cilantro for garnish (optional)

Instructions:

1. **Prepare the Tofu:** Drain the tofu and press it to remove excess moisture. You can use a tofu press or wrap the tofu in a clean kitchen towel and place a heavy object on top for about 20-30 minutes.

2. **Crumble the Tofu:** Once the tofu is drained, crumble it into small pieces using your hands or a fork. It should resemble the texture of scrambled eggs.

3. **Sauté the Vegetables:** Heat the olive oil in a large skillet over medium heat. Add the chopped onion and bell pepper. Sauté for about 3-5 minutes until they begin to soften.

4. **Add Tofu and Seasonings:** Add the crumbled tofu to the skillet. Sprinkle ground turmeric over the tofu for color and flavor. Season with salt and pepper to taste.

5. **Scramble and Cook:** Use a spatula to gently scramble the tofu and mix it with the sautéed vegetables. Cook for another 5-7 minutes, stirring occasionally, until the tofu is heated through and starts to develop a slightly golden color.

6. **Garnish and Serve:** Garnish your scrambled tofu with chopped fresh parsley or cilantro if desired.

Millet Porridge

Ingredients:

- 1/2 cup millet
- 2 cups water
- 1 1/2 cups low-fat or lactose-free milk (or a milk substitute like almond milk)
- 1-2 tablespoons honey or maple syrup (optional, for sweetness)
- 1/2 teaspoon vanilla extract (optional, for flavor)

- Soft fruit (e.g., mashed banana, cooked and mashed apples, or berries) for added flavor (optional)

- Chopped nuts (e.g., almonds or walnuts) for added texture (optional)

- A pinch of ground cinnamon (optional, for flavor)

- A pinch of salt (optional, for flavor)

Instructions:

1. **Rinse the Millet:** Place the millet in a fine-mesh strainer and rinse it thoroughly under cold running water. This helps remove any residual bitterness.

2. **Combine Millet and Water:** In a saucepan, combine the rinsed millet and 2 cups of water. Bring it to a boil over medium-high heat.

3. **Simmer the Millet:** Once it boils, reduce the heat to low, cover the saucepan with a lid, and let the millet simmer for about 15-20 minutes or until the grains are tender and have absorbed most of the water. Stir occasionally to prevent sticking.

4. **Add Milk:** Pour in the low-fat or lactose-free milk (or milk substitute) and stir to combine. Continue to cook over low heat.

5. **Sweeten and Flavor (Optional):**

- If desired, add honey or maple syrup for sweetness. Start with 1-2 tablespoons and adjust to your taste.
- You can also add vanilla extract for extra flavor.

- Optionally, add a pinch of ground cinnamon for a warm and comforting flavor.

6. **Add Soft Fruit (Optional):** To enhance the flavor and texture, consider adding soft fruits like mashed banana, cooked and mashed apples, or berries to the millet porridge. These fruits are generally gentle on the digestive system.

7. **Cook Until Desired Consistency:** Continue to cook the porridge, stirring occasionally, until it reaches your desired consistency. You can add more milk if you prefer a thinner porridge.

8. **Serve Warm:** Your millet porridge is now ready to be served. It should have a creamy and comforting texture.

9. **Enjoy:** Serve the millet porridge warm, and you can garnish it with chopped nuts

(e.g., almonds or walnuts) for added texture and flavor.

Slow Cooker Pork Bone Broth

Ingredients:

- 2-3 pounds pork bones (such as neck bones, marrow bones, or a combination)
- 1 onion, peeled and chopped
- 2 carrots, chopped
- 2 celery stalks, chopped
- 3-4 cloves garlic, crushed
- 2 bay leaves
- 1 teaspoon whole black peppercorns
- 1-2 tablespoons apple cider vinegar (helps extract minerals from the bones)
- 12 cups water (approximately)
- Salt to taste (add after cooking, if desired)

Instructions:

1. **Prep the Bones:** If your pork bones have any remaining bits of meat, you can brown them in the oven for added flavor. Place the bones on a baking sheet and roast them at 350°F (175°C) for about 30 minutes or until they develop a light brown color. This step is optional but can enhance the broth's flavor.

2. **Place Ingredients in Slow Cooker:** Place the roasted or unroasted pork bones in your slow cooker. Add the chopped onion, carrots, celery, crushed garlic, bay leaves, whole black peppercorns, and apple cider vinegar.

3. **Add Water:** Pour enough water into the slow cooker to cover the ingredients, typically about 12 cups of water, but adjust as needed to ensure everything is fully submerged.

4. **Cook on Low Heat:** Set your slow cooker to low heat and let the mixture simmer for 8-10 hours or overnight. Cooking it for an extended period helps extract the maximum flavor and nutrients from the bones.

5. **Strain the Broth:** Once the cooking time is complete, carefully strain the broth through a fine-mesh sieve or cheesecloth into another pot or container. Discard the solids or save them for another use.

6. **Season with Salt:** Taste the pork bone broth and season it with salt as desired. Add a little at a time, tasting between additions, until it reaches your preferred level of saltiness.

7. **Cool and Store:** Allow the broth to cool to room temperature before storing it in airtight containers. You can refrigerate it

for up to 4-5 days or freeze it for longer storage.

8. **Use in Recipes:** Use your homemade pork bone broth as a base for soups, stews, risottos, or any other recipes that call for broth. It will add rich flavor and nutrients to your dishes.

Rice Cake with Nut Butter

Ingredients:

- 2 rice cakes (choose plain, unsalted rice cakes)
- 2 tablespoons nut butter (e.g., almond butter, peanut butter, or sunflower seed butter)
- 1 small ripe banana, thinly sliced (optional, for added flavor and texture)
- A drizzle of honey or maple syrup (optional, for sweetness)

- A sprinkle of ground cinnamon (optional, for flavor)

Instructions:

1. Select Rice Cakes: Choose plain rice cakes that do not contain added salt or flavorings. These are gentler on the digestive system.

2. Spread Nut Butter: Take one rice cake and spread one tablespoon of your preferred nut butter (e.g., almond butter, peanut butter, or sunflower seed butter) evenly over its surface. You can use more or less nut butter depending on your preference.

3. **Add Banana Slices (Optional):** If you'd like to enhance the flavor and texture, place thinly sliced banana pieces on top of the nut butter.

4. **Drizzle Sweetener (Optional):** For added sweetness, drizzle a little honey or maple syrup over the banana slices. Adjust the amount to your taste.

5. **Sprinkle with Cinnamon (Optional):** Optionally, sprinkle a pinch of ground cinnamon over the top for extra flavor.

6. **Repeat for the Second Rice Cake:** Repeat the process for the second rice cake, spreading nut butter and adding optional toppings.

7. **Serve:** Your rice cakes with nut butter are now ready to be served. They make for a quick and satisfying snack or light meal.

Breakfast casseroles and frittatas

1. Breakfast Casserole for Diverticulitis:

Ingredients:

- 6 large eggs
- 1 cup lactose-free or low-fat milk (or a milk substitute)
- 2 cups diced cooked chicken or turkey (skinless and boneless)
- 1 cup cooked and diced potatoes
- 1 cup cooked and chopped spinach (or another soft leafy green)
- 1/2 cup grated cheddar cheese (optional)
- Salt and pepper to taste
- A pinch of ground paprika (optional, for flavor)

Instructions:

1. Preheat your oven to 350°F (175°C). Grease a baking dish (8x8 inches or similar size).

2. In a large bowl, whisk together the eggs and milk until well combined. Season with salt, pepper, and ground paprika if desired.

3. Add the diced cooked chicken or turkey, cooked potatoes, chopped spinach, and grated cheddar cheese (if using) to the egg mixture. Mix everything together.

4. Pour the mixture into the greased baking dish.

5. Bake in the preheated oven for approximately 30-35 minutes or until the casserole is set and the top is lightly golden.

6. Remove from the oven and let it cool for a few minutes before serving.

7. Slice and serve your breakfast casserole. It's a hearty and easy-to-digest option for a morning meal.

2. Spinach and Mushroom Frittata for Diverticulitis:

Ingredients:

- 6 large eggs
- 1/4 cup lactose-free or low-fat milk (or a milk substitute)
- 1 cup chopped spinach (cooked and drained)
- 1 cup sliced mushrooms
- 1/2 onion, finely chopped
- 1 clove garlic, minced
- 1/2 cup grated Parmesan cheese (optional)
- Salt and pepper to taste
- 1 tablespoon olive oil

Instructions:

1. Preheat your oven's broiler.

2. In an oven-safe skillet (cast iron works well), heat the olive oil over medium heat. Add the chopped onion and sliced mushrooms. Sauté for about 5-7 minutes until they are softened and any moisture from the mushrooms has evaporated.

3. Add the minced garlic and sauté for an additional minute until fragrant.

4. In a separate bowl, whisk together the eggs, milk, grated Parmesan cheese (if using), salt, and pepper.

5. Pour the egg mixture over the sautéed vegetables in the skillet. Stir gently to distribute the ingredients evenly.

6. Cook on the stovetop for 3-4 minutes until the edges start to set.

7. Transfer the skillet to the preheat broiler and cook for 2-3 minutes or until the frittata is set and the top is lightly golden.

8. Carefully remove the skillet from the oven (remember that the handle will be hot).

9. Let the frittata cool for a few minutes before slicing and serving.

Sweet potato hash with kale and turkey sausage

Ingredients:
- 2 large sweet potatoes, peeled and diced into small cubes
- 1 bunch of kale, stems removed and leaves chopped
- 8 ounces of lean turkey sausage, casings removed
- 1/2 onion, finely chopped

- 2 cloves garlic, minced
- 1/2 teaspoon paprika
- 1/2 teaspoon dried thyme
- Salt and pepper to taste
- Olive oil for cooking

Instructions:

1. **Pre Cook Sweet Potatoes:** Place the diced sweet potatoes in a microwave-safe bowl. Cover with a microwave-safe plate and cook in the microwave for about 3-4 minutes until they start to soften. This will reduce their cooking time in the skillet.

2. **Cook Turkey Sausage:** In a large skillet, heat a bit of olive oil over medium-high heat. Add the turkey sausage, breaking it up with a spoon, and cook until it's browned and cooked

through. Remove the cooked sausage from the skillet and set it aside.

3. **Sauté Onion and Garlic:** In the same skillet, add a little more olive oil if needed, then add the chopped onion and minced garlic. Sauté for about 2-3 minutes until they become fragrant and start to soften.

4. **Cook Sweet Potatoes:** Add the pre cooked sweet potato cubes to the skillet. Season with paprika, dried thyme, salt, and pepper. Stir to coat the sweet potatoes with the seasonings.

5. **Cook Kale:** Add the chopped kale to the skillet. It may seem like a lot at first, but it wilts down as it cooks. Stir everything together.

6. **Cover and Cook:** Cover the skillet with a lid and let the mixture cook for about 10-15 minutes, stirring occasionally,

until the sweet potatoes are tender and the kale is wilted and cooked down.

7. **Add Cooked Sausage:** Return the cooked turkey sausage to the skillet and stir it into the sweet potato and kale mixture. Cook for an additional 2-3 minutes to heat through.

8. **Serve:** Your sweet potato hash with kale and turkey sausage is now ready to be served. You can garnish it with a sprinkle of additional thyme or paprika if desired.

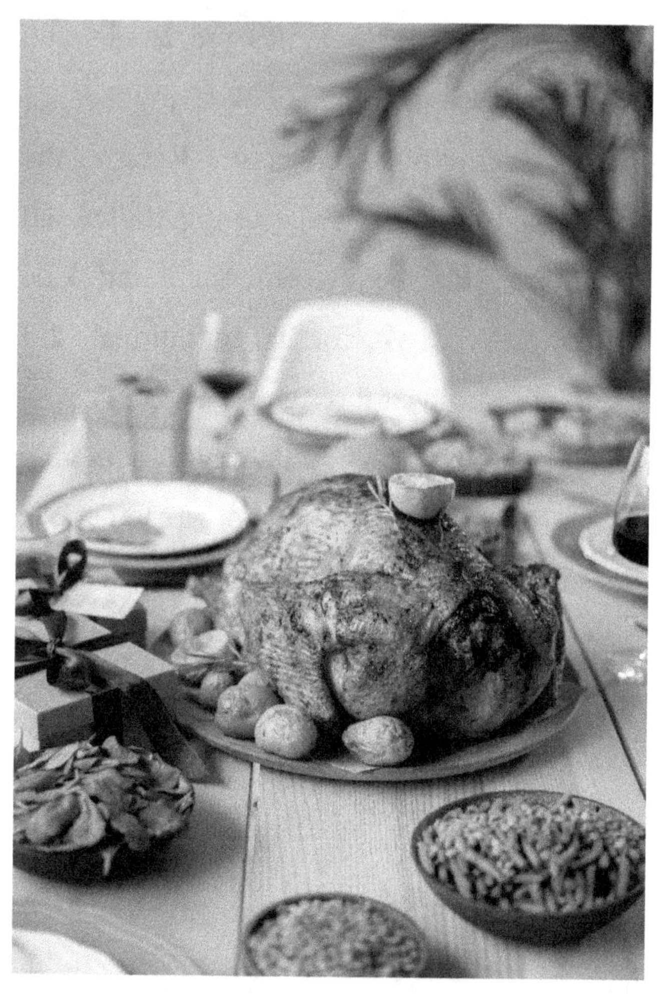

CHAPTER 3

LUNCH RECIPES

Grilled Chicken Salad:

Ingredients:

For the Grilled Chicken:

- 2 boneless, skinless chicken breasts
- 1 tablespoon olive oil
- 1 teaspoon dried thyme
- 1 teaspoon dried rosemary
- Salt and pepper to taste

For the Salad:

- 6 cups mixed greens (e.g., lettuce, spinach, arugula)
- 1 cup cherry tomatoes, halved
- 1 cucumber, sliced
- 1/2 red onion, thinly sliced

- 1/4 cup Kalamata olives, pitted and sliced (optional, if tolerated)
- 1/4 cup feta cheese, crumbled (optional, if tolerated)

For the Dressing:

- 3 tablespoons extra-virgin olive oil
- 2 tablespoons balsamic vinegar
- 1 teaspoon Dijon mustard
- 1 clove garlic, minced
- Salt and pepper to taste

Instructions:

1. **Prepare the Grilled Chicken:**
- Preheat your grill or grill pan over medium-high heat.
- In a small bowl, mix together the olive oil, dried thyme, dried rosemary, salt, and pepper.

- Brush the chicken breasts with the herb-infused olive oil mixture.

- Grill the chicken breasts for about 6-8 minutes per side or until they are cooked through and have nice grill marks. The internal temperature should reach 165°F (74°C).

- Remove the chicken from the grill and let it rest for a few minutes before slicing it into thin strips.

2. **Make the Salad:** In a large salad bowl, combine the mixed greens, cherry tomatoes, cucumber slices, red onion, and Kalamata olives (if using). Toss gently to mix the ingredients.

3. **Prepare the Dressing:** In a small bowl, whisk together the extra-virgin olive oil, balsamic vinegar, Dijon mustard, minced garlic, salt, and pepper until well combined.

4. **Assemble the Salad:**

- Place the sliced grilled chicken on top of the salad.

- If you tolerate feta cheese, sprinkle it over the salad.

- Drizzle the dressing over the salad just before serving.

5. **Serve:**

- Toss the salad gently to coat all the ingredients with the dressing.

- Serve your grilled chicken salad as a nutritious and satisfying meal.

Quinoa and Vegetable Bowl:

Ingredients:

For the Quinoa:

- 1 cup quinoa

- 2 cups water or low-sodium vegetable broth

- Salt (optional)

For the Vegetables:

- 2 cups mixed vegetables (e.g., bell peppers, zucchini, cherry tomatoes, broccoli, carrots, etc.), chopped into bite-sized pieces
- 2 tablespoons olive oil
- Salt and pepper to taste
- Dried herbs or spices of your choice (e.g., thyme, oregano, paprika, or cumin)

For the Dressing:

- 3 tablespoons extra-virgin olive oil
- 1-2 tablespoons balsamic vinegar or lemon juice
- 1 clove garlic, minced
- Salt and pepper to taste

Optional Toppings:

- Sliced avocado

- Chopped fresh herbs (e.g., parsley, cilantro, or basil)

- Crumbled feta cheese (if tolerated)

- Nuts or seeds (e.g., almonds, pumpkin seeds, or sunflower seeds)

Instructions:

1. **Cook the Quinoa:**

- Rinse the quinoa thoroughly in a fine-mesh strainer under cold running water to remove any bitterness.

- In a medium saucepan, combine the rinsed quinoa, water (or vegetable broth), and a pinch of salt if desired. Bring it to a boil over medium-high heat.

- Reduce the heat to low, cover the saucepan with a lid, and let the quinoa simmer for about 15-20 minutes, or until all the liquid is absorbed and the quinoa is fluffy. Remove from heat and fluff with a fork.

2. **Roast the Vegetables:**

- Preheat your oven to 425°F (220°C).

- In a large mixing bowl, toss the chopped mixed vegetables with olive oil, salt, pepper, and your choice of dried herbs or spices.

- Spread the seasoned vegetables in a single layer on a baking sheet.

- Roast the vegetables in the preheated oven for about 20-25 minutes or until they are tender and slightly caramelized. Stir them once or twice during roasting to ensure even cooking.

3. **Prepare the Dressing:** In a small bowl, whisk together the extra-virgin olive oil, balsamic vinegar or lemon juice, minced garlic, salt, and pepper. Adjust the quantities to your taste.

4. **Assemble the Bowl:**

- Divide the cooked quinoa among serving bowls.

- Top the quinoa with the roasted vegetables.

- Drizzle the dressing over the vegetables and quinoa.

5. **Add Optional Toppings:** If desired, garnish your quinoa and vegetable bowl with sliced avocado, chopped fresh herbs, crumbled feta cheese (if tolerated), or nuts/seeds for added texture and flavor.

6. **Serve:** Your quinoa and vegetable bowl is now ready to be served. Enjoy it as a wholesome and satisfying meal.

Turkey and Avocado Wrap:

Ingredients:

- 1 large whole wheat or gluten-free tortilla wrap (choose one suitable for your dietary needs)
- 4-6 slices of lean turkey breast
- 1/2 ripe avocado, sliced
- 1/4 cup shredded lettuce or baby spinach
- 2-3 slices of tomato
- 2-3 slices of cucumber
- 1-2 tablespoons hummus or Greek yogurt (as a spread, optional)
- Salt and pepper to taste
- A squeeze of fresh lemon juice (optional, for added flavor)

Instructions:

1. **Prepare the Tortilla Wrap:** Lay the tortilla wrap flat on a clean surface or a large plate.

2. **Add a Spread (Optional):** If you prefer, spread a thin layer of hummus or Greek yogurt over the center of the tortilla. This will add flavor and help hold the ingredients together.

3. **Layer the Ingredients:**

- Place the turkey slices in the center of the tortilla, slightly overlapping them.

- Arrange the avocado slices, shredded lettuce or baby spinach, tomato slices, and cucumber slices evenly over the turkey.

- Season the ingredients with a pinch of salt and pepper. For extra flavor, you can also squeeze a bit of fresh lemon juice over the vegetables.

4. **Fold and Roll:**

- Carefully fold in the sides of the tortilla to cover the ingredients.

- Starting from the bottom, tightly roll up the tortilla, enclosing all the fillings.

5. **Cut and Serve:**

- Using a sharp knife, cut the turkey and avocado wrap in half diagonally.

- Serve immediately, or you can wrap it in parchment paper or foil for a portable meal.

6. **Enjoy:** Your turkey and avocado wrap is ready to enjoy as a satisfying and balanced meal.

Greek Yogurt Tuna Salad:

Ingredients:

- 1 can (5-6 ounces) of tuna in water, drained
- 1/2 cup Greek yogurt (plain, low-fat, or non-fat)
- 2 tablespoons mayonnaise (optional, for extra creaminess)
- 1 celery stalk, finely chopped
- 1/4 red onion, finely chopped
- 1/4 cup diced cucumber
- 1/4 cup diced red bell pepper
- 1/4 cup diced carrots
- 1 tablespoon fresh lemon juice
- 1 tablespoon fresh dill, chopped (or 1 teaspoon dried dill)
- Salt and pepper to taste
- Lettuce leaves or whole wheat bread (for serving)

Instructions:

1. **Prepare the Tuna:**

- Open the can of tuna and drain the water or oil.

- Place the drained tuna in a mixing bowl and use a fork to break it into smaller flakes.

2. **Add Greek Yogurt:** Add the Greek yogurt to the bowl with the tuna. If you prefer a creamier salad, you can also add mayonnaise at this point.

3. **Mix in Vegetables:** Add the chopped celery, red onion, cucumber, red bell pepper, and carrots to the bowl with the tuna and Greek yogurt.

4. **Season and Flavor:**

- Squeeze fresh lemon juice over the salad to add a fresh and tangy flavor.

- Sprinkle fresh dill over the mixture. If you don't have fresh dill, you can use dried dill.

5. **Season with Salt and Pepper:** Season the salad with salt and pepper to taste. Start with a little, and you can always add more if needed.

6. **Mix Thoroughly:** Use a spoon to thoroughly mix all the ingredients together until the tuna and vegetables are evenly coated with the Greek yogurt mixture.

7. **Serve:**

- You can serve Greek yogurt tuna salad in various ways:

- As a sandwich: Spoon the salad onto whole wheat bread or a roll and top it with lettuce leaves.

- As a lettuce wrap: Scoop the salad into lettuce leaves and roll them up.

- On a bed of greens: Serve the salad on a bed of lettuce, spinach, or mixed greens for a lighter option.

- With crackers: Enjoy it with whole-grain crackers or rice cakes.

8. **Enjoy:** Your Greek yogurt tuna salad is now ready to enjoy as a healthy and protein-rich meal or snack.

Egg Salad Sandwich:

Ingredients:

- 4 large eggs
- 2-3 tablespoons mayonnaise (use a low-fat or olive oil-based mayo for a lighter option)
- 1 teaspoon Dijon mustard
- 1/4 cup finely chopped celery
- 2 tablespoons finely chopped red onion (you can use scallions or green onions as a milder alternative)
- Salt and pepper to taste

- Whole wheat bread or your preferred bread (choose one that's gentle on your digestive system)
- Lettuce leaves (optional, for added texture and flavor)

Instructions:

1. **Hard-Boil the Eggs:**

- Place the eggs in a saucepan and cover them with cold water.
- Bring the water to a boil over medium-high heat.
- Once it boils, remove the saucepan from the heat, cover it with a lid, and let the eggs sit in the hot water for about 9-12 minutes to hard-boil.
- Drain the hot water and transfer the eggs to a bowl of ice water to cool quickly. This will make peeling the eggs easier.

2. **Peel and Chop the Eggs:** Once the eggs are cool, peel them and chop them finely. You can use an egg slicer or a knife to achieve your preferred consistency, whether you like a chunkier or smoother egg salad.

3. **Make the Egg Salad:**

- In a mixing bowl, combine the chopped eggs, mayonnaise, Dijon mustard, chopped celery, and chopped red onion.

- Season with salt and pepper to taste. Start with a little salt and pepper and adjust to your preference.

4. **Mix Thoroughly:** Use a spoon to mix all the ingredients together until well combined and the egg salad has a creamy consistency.

5. **Assemble the Sandwich:** Spread the egg salad generously onto slices of whole wheat bread. You can add lettuce leaves

for added texture and freshness if desired.

6. **Serve:** Your egg salad sandwich is now ready to be served. Pair it with a side of fresh vegetables or a simple salad for a complete meal.

Butternut Squash Soup:

Ingredients:

- 1 medium-sized butternut squash, peeled, seeded, and diced (approximately 4 cups)
- 1 onion, chopped
- 2 cloves garlic, minced
- 2 carrots, peeled and chopped
- 2 celery stalks, chopped
- 1 apple, peeled, cored, and chopped (optional, for sweetness)
- 4 cups low-sodium vegetable broth
- 1 teaspoon olive oil
- 1 teaspoon dried thyme

- 1/2 teaspoon ground cinnamon

- Salt and pepper to taste

- Optional garnishes: Greek yogurt or sour cream, chopped fresh herbs (e.g., parsley or chives), croutons, or roasted pumpkin seeds

Instructions:

1. **Prepare the Butternut Squash:** Peel the butternut squash, remove the seeds, and dice it into small pieces. Set aside.

2. **Sauté Onions and Garlic:**

- In a large soup pot, heat the olive oil over medium heat.

- Add the chopped onion and minced garlic. Sauté for about 2-3 minutes until they become fragrant and slightly softened.

3. **Add Vegetables:** Add the chopped carrots, celery, and apple (if using) to the

pot. Sauté for an additional 5-6 minutes until the vegetables start to soften.

4. **Season:**

- Sprinkle the dried thyme and ground cinnamon over the sautéed vegetables.

- Season with salt and pepper to taste. Start with a little and adjust later if needed.

5. **Cook the Squash:**

- Add the diced butternut squash to the pot and stir everything together.

- Pour in the low-sodium vegetable broth to cover the vegetables and squash.

6. **Simmer:** Bring the mixture to a boil, then reduce the heat to low. Cover the pot with a lid and let it simmer for about 20-25 minutes or until the vegetables and butternut squash are tender.

7. **Blend the Soup:** Use an immersion blender to puree the soup directly in the

pot until it's smooth and creamy. If you don't have an immersion blender, carefully transfer the soup in batches to a regular blender and blend until smooth. Be cautious as hot soup can splatter.

8. **Adjust Consistency:** If the soup is too thick for your liking, you can add a bit more vegetable broth to reach your desired consistency.

9. **Taste and Adjust Seasoning:** Taste the soup and adjust the seasoning with salt and pepper as needed.

10. **Serve:**

- Ladle the butternut squash soup into bowls.
- Garnish with a dollop of Greek yogurt or sour cream, chopped fresh herbs, croutons, or roasted pumpkin seeds, if desired.

11. **Enjoy:** Your butternut squash soup is now ready to be enjoyed as a comforting and nutritious meal.

Sweet Potato and Lentil Stew:

Ingredients:

- 1 cup dried green or brown lentils, rinsed and drained
- 2 medium sweet potatoes, peeled and diced
- 1 onion, chopped
- 2 carrots, peeled and chopped
- 2 celery stalks, chopped
- 2 cloves garlic, minced
- 1 can (14 ounces) diced tomatoes (preferably no-salt-added)
- 4 cups low-sodium vegetable broth
- 1 teaspoon ground cumin
- 1/2 teaspoon ground turmeric
- 1/2 teaspoon paprika

- Salt and pepper to taste

- Olive oil for sautéing

- Chopped fresh parsley (optional, for garnish)

Instructions:

1. **Sauté the Vegetables:**

- Heat a large soup pot over medium heat and add a drizzle of olive oil.

- Add the chopped onion, carrots, and celery. Sauté for about 5-7 minutes until the vegetables start to soften.

2. **Add Garlic and Spices:** Add the minced garlic, ground cumin, ground turmeric, and paprika to the pot. Sauté for an additional minute until the spices become fragrant.

3. **Add Lentils and Sweet Potatoes:** Add the rinsed and drained lentils and the diced sweet potatoes to the pot. Stir to

combine with the sautéed vegetables and spices.

4. **Pour in Tomatoes and Broth:**

- Pour in the can of diced tomatoes (including the juice) and the low-sodium vegetable broth.

- Season with salt and pepper to taste. Start with a little and adjust later if needed.

5. **Simmer:** Bring the mixture to a boil, then reduce the heat to low. Cover the pot with a lid and let the stew simmer for about 25-30 minutes or until the lentils and sweet potatoes are tender.

6. **Taste and Adjust Seasoning:** Taste the stew and adjust the seasoning with additional salt and pepper if necessary.

7. **Serve:**

- Ladle the sweet potato and lentil stew into bowls.

- Garnish with chopped fresh parsley if desired.

8. **Enjoy:** Your sweet potato and lentil stew is now ready to be enjoyed as a hearty and nourishing meal.

Roasted Vegetable Quiche:

Ingredients:

For the Pie Crust:

- 1 pre-made pie crust (store-bought or homemade)

For the Roasted Vegetables:

- 2 cups of assorted vegetables (e.g., bell peppers, zucchini, cherry tomatoes, broccoli, onions, etc.), chopped into small pieces

- 2 tablespoons olive oil
- Salt and pepper to taste
- Optional herbs or seasonings (e.g., dried thyme, rosemary, or paprika)

For the Quiche Filling:

- 4 large eggs
- 1 cup milk (use regular milk, lactose-free, or plant-based milk)
- 1/2 cup shredded cheese (e.g., cheddar, Swiss, or mozzarella)
- Salt and pepper to taste
- A pinch of nutmeg (optional, for added flavor)

Instructions:

1. **Roast the Vegetables:**

- Preheat your oven to 400°F (200°C).

- In a large bowl, toss the chopped vegetables with olive oil, salt, pepper, and any optional herbs or seasonings you prefer.

- Spread the seasoned vegetables in a single layer on a baking sheet.

- Roast in the preheated oven for approximately 20-25 minutes or until the vegetables are tender and slightly caramelized. Stir them once or twice during roasting to ensure even cooking.

- Remove the roasted vegetables from the oven and set them aside to cool slightly.

2. **Prepare the Pie Crust:**

- Preheat your oven to 375°F (190°C).

- Place the pre-made pie crust in a pie dish and press it down gently to fit the bottom and sides. You can also use a pie crust that you've made from scratch.

3. **Make the Quiche Filling:** In a mixing bowl, whisk together the eggs, milk, shredded cheese, salt, pepper, and a pinch of nutmeg (if using).

4. **Assemble the Quiche:**

- Arrange the roasted vegetables evenly over the bottom of the pie crust.

- Pour the quiche filling over the roasted vegetables.

5. **Bake:** Place the quiche in the preheated oven and bake for approximately 35-40 minutes, or until the quiche is set and the top is golden brown. You can insert a knife into the center; if it comes out clean, the quiche is done.

6. **Cool and Serve:** Allow the quiche to cool for a few minutes before slicing and serving. It can be served warm or at room temperature.

7. **Enjoy:** Your roasted vegetable quiche is now ready to be enjoyed as a delicious and satisfying meal.

Mashed Cauliflower:

Ingredients:

- 1 head of cauliflower, cut into florets
- 2 cloves garlic, minced
- 2 tablespoons olive oil or butter (choose one that suits your dietary needs)
- 1/4 cup low-sodium vegetable broth (or more for desired consistency)
- Salt and pepper to taste
- Chopped fresh herbs (e.g., parsley or chives, optional, for garnish)

Instructions:

1. **Steam the Cauliflower:**
- Place the cauliflower florets in a steamer basket over a pot of simmering water.

- Cover and steam for about 10-12 minutes or until the cauliflower is tender and can be easily pierced with a fork.

2. **Sauté Garlic:**

- While the cauliflower is steaming, heat the olive oil or butter in a small skillet over medium-low heat.

- Add the minced garlic and sauté for about 1-2 minutes until fragrant. Be careful not to brown or burn the garlic.

3. **Blend the Cauliflower:**

- Transfer the steamed cauliflower to a food processor or blender.

- Add the sautéed garlic and any residual oil or butter from the skillet.

- Start with 1/4 cup of low-sodium vegetable broth and add it to the blender.

- Blend until smooth and creamy, adding more vegetable broth as needed to reach your desired consistency. The mixture should be similar to mashed potatoes.

4. **Season:** Season the mashed cauliflower with salt and pepper to taste. Start with a little and adjust to your preference.

5. **Serve:**

- Transfer the mashed cauliflower to a serving dish.

- If desired, garnish with chopped fresh herbs, such as parsley or chives.

6. **Enjoy:** Your mashed cauliflower is now ready to be enjoyed as a nutritious and diverticulitis-friendly side dish.

Turkey and Rice Soup:

Ingredients:

- 2 cups cooked turkey (light meat or a mix of light and dark meat), shredded or diced

- 1 cup white or brown rice, cooked

- 1 onion, chopped

- 2 carrots, peeled and diced

- 2 celery stalks, diced

- 2 cloves garlic, minced

- 8 cups low-sodium chicken or turkey broth

- 1 bay leaf

- 1 teaspoon dried thyme

- Salt and pepper to taste

- Olive oil for sautéing

- Chopped fresh parsley (optional, for garnish)

Instructions:

1. **Sauté the Vegetables:**

- In a large soup pot, heat a drizzle of olive oil over medium heat.

- Add the chopped onion, diced carrots, and diced celery. Sauté for about 5-7 minutes until the vegetables begin to soften.

2. **Add Garlic and Seasonings:** Stir in the minced garlic, dried thyme, and the bay leaf. Sauté for an additional minute until the garlic becomes fragrant.

3. **Pour in Broth:** Add the low-sodium chicken or turkey broth to the pot. You can use store-bought or homemade broth.

4. **Bring to a Boil:** Bring the broth to a boil, then reduce the heat to low and let it simmer for about 10-15 minutes to allow the flavors to meld.

5. **Add Turkey and Rice:** Add the cooked turkey and cooked rice to the simmering soup. Stir to combine.

6. **Simmer:** Let the soup simmer for an additional 10-15 minutes to heat the turkey and rice thoroughly.

7. **Season:** Season the soup with salt and pepper to taste. Start with a little and adjust to your preference.

8. **Remove Bay Leaf:** Don't forget to remove the bay leaf before serving. It's for flavoring and not meant to be eaten.

9. **Serve:** Ladle the turkey and rice soup into bowls.

10. **Garnish (Optional):** If desired, garnish the soup with chopped fresh parsley for a burst of freshness and color.

11. **Enjoy:** Your turkey and rice soup is now ready to be enjoyed as a comforting and diverticulitis-friendly meal.

Grilled Shrimp Skewers:

Ingredients:

- 1 pound large shrimp, peeled and deveined
- 2 tablespoons olive oil

- 2 cloves garlic, minced

- 1 teaspoon paprika

- 1/2 teaspoon dried oregano

- 1/2 teaspoon dried thyme

- Salt and pepper to taste

- Wooden skewers, soaked in water for at least 30 minutes to prevent burning

- Lemon wedges (for serving, optional)

Instructions:

1. **Marinate the Shrimp:**

- In a mixing bowl, combine the olive oil, minced garlic, paprika, dried oregano, dried thyme, salt, and pepper. Mix well to create a marinade.

- Add the peeled and deveined shrimp to the marinade, and toss to coat them evenly. Cover the bowl and refrigerate for at least 15-30 minutes to allow the flavors to meld.

2. **Preheat the Grill:** Preheat your grill to medium-high heat, around 350-400°F (175-200°C).

3. **Skewer the Shrimp:** Thread the marinated shrimp onto the soaked wooden skewers. Make sure to leave a small gap between each shrimp to ensure even cooking.

4. **Grill the Shrimp:**

- Place the shrimp skewers on the preheated grill.

- Grill for about 2-3 minutes per side or until the shrimp turn pink and opaque. Be cautious not to overcook them, as shrimp can become tough when overdone.

5. **Serve:**

- Remove the grilled shrimp skewers from the grill.

- Serve them hot with lemon wedges for a burst of citrus flavor if desired.

6. **Enjoy:** Your grilled shrimp skewers are now ready to be enjoyed as a flavorful and protein-rich meal.

Sautéed Spinach and Mushrooms:

Ingredients:

- 8 ounces fresh spinach leaves, washed and stemmed
- 8 ounces mushrooms, sliced
- 2 cloves garlic, minced
- 2 tablespoons olive oil
- Salt and pepper to taste
- A pinch of red pepper flakes (optional, for added heat)
- Fresh lemon juice (optional, for a zesty finish)

Instructions:

1. **Prep the Spinach:** Wash the fresh spinach leaves thoroughly and remove any tough stems. You can leave the tender stems attached.

2. **Sauté the Mushrooms:**

- Heat the olive oil in a large skillet over medium-high heat.

- Add the sliced mushrooms to the skillet and sauté them for about 5-7 minutes, or until they become tender and start to release their moisture.

3. **Add Garlic and Spinach:**

- Add the minced garlic to the skillet with the mushrooms and sauté for an additional 1-2 minutes until fragrant.

- Gradually add the fresh spinach leaves to the skillet, a handful at a time. As the spinach wilts, you can add more until all the spinach is in the pan.

- Continue to sauté the spinach and mushrooms together for 2-3 minutes until the spinach is wilted but still bright green.

4. **Season:** Season the sautéed spinach and mushrooms with salt, pepper, and a pinch of red pepper flakes if you desire a bit of heat.

5. **Finish with Lemon Juice (Optional):** For a zesty touch, squeeze fresh lemon juice over the sautéed spinach and mushrooms just before serving.

6. **Serve:** Transfer the sautéed spinach and mushrooms to a serving dish.

7. **Enjoy:** Your sautéed spinach and mushrooms are now ready to be enjoyed as a flavorful and nutrient-packed side dish.

Tofu Stir-Fry:

Ingredients:

For the Tofu:

- 14 ounces (400g) firm tofu, cubed
- 2 tablespoons low-sodium soy sauce (or tamari for a gluten-free option)
- 1 teaspoon sesame oil
- 1 teaspoon olive oil or vegetable oil for cooking

For the Stir-Fry:

- 2 cups mixed vegetables (e.g., bell peppers, broccoli, carrots, snap peas, or any of your favorites), sliced or chopped
- 2 cloves garlic, minced
- 1-inch piece of ginger, minced or grated
- 2 tablespoons low-sodium soy sauce (or tamari)

- 1 tablespoon olive oil or vegetable oil for cooking
- Salt and pepper to taste
- Cooked brown rice or whole grain rice (for serving)

Instructions:

1. **Marinate the Tofu:** In a mixing bowl, combine the cubed tofu, 2 tablespoons of low-sodium soy sauce, and 1 teaspoon of sesame oil. Gently toss the tofu to coat it with the marinade. Set it aside to marinate while you prepare the rest of the ingredients.

2. **Prepare the Vegetables:** Slice or chop the mixed vegetables of your choice. Keep them uniform in size for even cooking.

3. **Sauté the Tofu:**

- Heat 1 teaspoon of olive oil or vegetable oil in a large skillet or wok over medium-high heat.

- Add the marinated tofu cubes to the skillet, ensuring they are in a single layer. Cook for about 2-3 minutes per side, or until they are golden brown and slightly crispy. Remove the tofu from the skillet and set it aside.

4. **Sauté the Vegetables:**

- In the same skillet, add the remaining 1 tablespoon of oil.

- Add the minced garlic and ginger, and sauté for about 30 seconds until fragrant.

- Add the chopped vegetables to the skillet and stir-fry for about 4-5 minutes, or until they are tender-crisp.

5. **Combine Tofu and Vegetables:** Return the cooked tofu to the skillet with the sautéed vegetables.

6. **Add Soy Sauce:** Drizzle 2 tablespoons of low-sodium soy sauce (or tamari) over the tofu and vegetables. Stir-fry for an additional 1-2 minutes to heat everything through and allow the flavors to meld.

7. **Season:** Season the tofu stir-fry with salt and pepper to taste. Adjust the seasonings as needed.

8. **Serve:** Serve the tofu stir-fry hot over cooked brown rice or whole grain rice.

9. **Enjoy:** Your tofu stir-fry is now ready to be enjoyed as a wholesome and diverticulitis-friendly meal.

Zucchini Noodles:

Ingredients:

- 2-3 medium-sized zucchinis

- Olive oil

- Salt and pepper to taste

- Optional toppings: grated Parmesan cheese, chopped fresh herbs, or your favorite pasta sauce (ensure it's low in seeds and high in fiber)

Instructions:

1. **Prepare the Zucchinis:**

- Wash the zucchinis thoroughly under running water.

- Trim the ends of the zucchinis.

- Depending on your preference, you can leave the skin on or peel it off. Leaving the skin on adds extra fiber and nutrients.

- Cut the zucchinis into noodles using a spiralizer, julienne peeler, or a knife. The thickness of the noodles is up to you, but thinner noodles tend to cook faster.

2. **Sauté the Zucchini Noodles:**

- Heat a large skillet over medium-high heat and add a drizzle of olive oil.

- Once the oil is hot, add the zucchini noodles to the skillet.

- Sauté the noodles for 2-3 minutes, stirring frequently, until they begin to soften. Be careful not to overcook; zucchini noodles should remain slightly crisp.

3. **Season:** Season the zucchini noodles with salt and pepper to taste. Keep it simple to avoid potential irritants.

4. **Serve:** Transfer the sautéed zucchini noodles to a serving plate.

5. **Add Toppings (Optional):** If desired, you can top the zucchini noodles with grated Parmesan cheese, chopped fresh herbs (e.g., basil or parsley), or a diverticulitis-friendly pasta sauce.

6. **Enjoy:** Your zucchini noodles are now ready to be enjoyed as a healthy and diverticulitis-friendly alternative to traditional pasta.

Baked Chicken and Rice:

Ingredients:

- 4 boneless, skinless chicken breasts
- 1 cup long-grain white rice
- 2 cups low-sodium chicken broth
- 1 onion, chopped
- 2 cloves garlic, minced
- 1 cup mixed vegetables (e.g., carrots, peas, green beans)
- 2 tablespoons olive oil
- 1 teaspoon dried thyme
- Salt and pepper to taste
- Lemon wedges (optional, for serving)

Instructions:

1. **Preheat the Oven:** Preheat your oven to 375°F (190°C).

2. **Sauté the Vegetables:**

- In a large ovenproof skillet or baking dish, heat the olive oil over medium heat.

- Add the chopped onion and minced garlic, and sauté for about 2-3 minutes until they become fragrant and slightly softened.

- Stir in the mixed vegetables and cook for an additional 2-3 minutes.

3. **Add Rice and Seasonings:**

- Add the white rice to the skillet with the sautéed vegetables. Stir to combine.

- Sprinkle the dried thyme, salt, and pepper over the rice mixture, and stir to distribute the seasonings evenly.

4. **Arrange the Chicken:** Place the boneless, skinless chicken breasts on top

of the rice mixture in the skillet or baking dish.

5. **Pour Chicken Broth:** Pour the low-sodium chicken broth evenly over the chicken and rice.

6. **Cover and Bake:**

- Cover the skillet or baking dish with a lid or aluminum foil.

- Place it in the preheated oven and bake for approximately 35-45 minutes or until the chicken is cooked through and the rice is tender. Cooking times may vary depending on your oven, so check for doneness by ensuring the chicken reaches an internal temperature of 165°F (74°C) and the rice is fully cooked.

7. **Serve:** Once done, remove the skillet or baking dish from the oven.

8. **Optional Lemon Wedges:** If desired, serve the baked chicken and rice with lemon wedges for a zesty finish.

9. **Enjoy:** Your baked chicken and rice is now ready to be enjoyed as a comforting and diverticulitis-friendly meal.

Lentil and Spinach Salad:

Ingredients:

For the Salad:

- 1 cup dried green or brown lentils, rinsed and drained
- 4 cups fresh spinach leaves, washed and stemmed
- 1/2 red onion, finely chopped
- 1 cucumber, diced
- 1 cup cherry tomatoes, halved
- 1/4 cup crumbled feta cheese (optional)
- 1/4 cup chopped fresh parsley or cilantro (optional, for garnish)

For the Dressing:

- 3 tablespoons extra-virgin olive oil
- 2 tablespoons red wine vinegar
- 1 clove garlic, minced
- 1/2 teaspoon Dijon mustard
- Salt and pepper to taste

Instructions:

1. Cook the Lentils:

- In a medium saucepan, combine the rinsed lentils with enough water to cover them by about 2 inches.
- Bring the water to a boil, then reduce the heat to a simmer and cook for 20-25 minutes or until the lentils are tender but not mushy.
- Drain any excess water and set the cooked lentils aside to cool.

2. **Prepare the Dressing:** In a small bowl, whisk together the extra-virgin olive oil, red wine vinegar, minced garlic, Dijon mustard, salt, and pepper. Set aside.

3. **Assemble the Salad:**

- In a large salad bowl, combine the cooked lentils, fresh spinach leaves, finely chopped red onion, diced cucumber, and halved cherry tomatoes.

- If desired, add crumbled feta cheese for extra flavor and creaminess.

4. **Add the Dressing:** Pour the dressing over the salad ingredients.

5. **Toss and Garnish:**

- Gently toss the salad to ensure all the ingredients are coated with the dressing.

- If desired, garnish the lentil and spinach salad with chopped fresh parsley or cilantro for a burst of freshness.

6. **Serve:** Serve the salad immediately as a
light and nutritious meal.

CHAPTER 4

DINNER

Baked Chicken Breast:

Ingredients:

- 2 boneless, skinless chicken breasts
- 1 tablespoon olive oil
- 1/2 teaspoon salt (or to taste)
- 1/4 teaspoon black pepper (or to taste)
- 1/2 teaspoon dried thyme (optional, for flavor)
- 1/2 teaspoon dried oregano (optional, for flavor)
- 1/2 teaspoon garlic powder (optional, for flavor)
- 1/2 teaspoon paprika (optional, for flavor)
- 1 lemon, sliced (optional, for added flavor)

- 1/4 cup low-sodium chicken broth (optional, for moisture)

Instructions:

1. **Preheat the Oven:** Preheat your oven to 375°F (190°C).

2. **Prepare the Chicken:** Rinse the chicken breasts under cold water and pat them dry with paper towels. This helps remove any potential contaminants. Place the chicken breasts on a clean cutting board.

3. **Season the Chicken:** Drizzle the olive oil over both sides of the chicken breasts. Season the chicken with salt and pepper. If you want to add more flavor, sprinkle on the dried thyme, oregano, garlic powder, and paprika. Gently rub the seasonings into the chicken to coat evenly.

4. **Place in Baking Dish:** If you're concerned about moisture, place the lemon slices on the bottom of a baking dish to prevent sticking. Place the seasoned chicken breasts on top of the lemon slices. You can also add the chicken broth to the bottom of the dish for extra moisture if desired.

5. **Bake:** Cover the baking dish with aluminum foil to help trap moisture. Bake in the preheated oven for approximately 25-30 minutes, or until the chicken reaches an internal temperature of 165°F (74°C). Cooking time may vary depending on the thickness of your chicken breasts, so use a meat thermometer to ensure they are cooked thoroughly.

6. **Rest and Serve:** Once cooked, remove the chicken from the oven and let it rest

for a few minutes before slicing. This allows the juices to redistribute and keeps the chicken moist. Serve with your choice of cooked vegetables or a simple mashed potato if your diverticulitis permits.

Herb-Crusted Baked Cod:

Ingredients:

- 2 cod filets (about 6 ounces each)
- 2 tablespoons plain breadcrumbs (make sure they don't contain seeds)
- 1 tablespoon fresh parsley, chopped
- 1 teaspoon dried thyme (or other preferred herbs)
- 1/2 teaspoon salt (or to taste)
- 1/4 teaspoon black pepper (or to taste)
- 1 tablespoon olive oil
- 1 lemon, sliced for garnish (optional)

Instructions:

1. **Preheat the Oven:** Preheat your oven to 375°F (190°C).

2. **Prepare the Cod:** Rinse the cod filets under cold water and pat them dry with paper towels. Place the cod filets on a clean plate or cutting board.

3. **Prepare the Herb Crust:** In a small bowl, combine the breadcrumbs, chopped parsley, dried thyme, salt, and black pepper. Mix well to create the herb crust mixture.

4. **Coat the Cod:** Brush each cod filet lightly with olive oil, ensuring they are evenly coated. Then, press the herb crust mixture onto both sides of the cod filets. The coating should adhere nicely.

5. **Bake:** Place the coated cod fillets on a baking sheet lined with parchment paper

to prevent sticking. If desired, you can place lemon slices on top of the filets for added flavor and moisture. Bake in the preheated oven for about 15-20 minutes, or until the cod is opaque and flakes easily with a fork. Cooking time may vary depending on the thickness of the filets.

6. **Rest and Serve:** Once the cod is cooked, remove it from the oven and let it rest for a couple of minutes. This allows the juices to settle, keeping the fish moist. Serve the herb-crusted baked cod with steamed or mashed potatoes and steamed vegetables for a well-balanced meal.

Turkey and Rice Soup:

Ingredients:

- 1 cup cooked turkey breast, shredded (skinless and boneless)
- 1/2 cup white rice, rinsed and drained
- 4 cups low-sodium chicken broth (homemade or store-bought)
- 1 carrot, peeled and diced
- 1 celery stalk, diced
- 1/2 cup cooked and diced zucchini (optional)
- 1/2 teaspoon dried thyme
- Salt and pepper to taste
- Chopped fresh parsley for garnish (optional)

Instructions:

1. **Prepare the Rice:** In a small saucepan, cook the white rice according to the package instructions. Set it aside when it's cooked.

2. **Cook the Vegetables:** In a large soup pot, heat a bit of olive oil over medium heat. Add the diced carrot and celery. Sauté for a few minutes until they start to soften.

3. **Add the Turkey and Broth:** Add the shredded turkey breast to the pot with the sautéed vegetables. Pour in the low-sodium chicken broth.

4. **Season and Simmer:** Season the soup with dried thyme, salt, and pepper. Bring the mixture to a boil, then reduce the heat to low, cover the pot, and let it simmer for about 10-15 minutes, or until the vegetables are tender.

5. **Add Cooked Rice:** Once the vegetables are tender, add the cooked rice to the soup. If you have cooked and diced zucchini, you can add it now as well. Allow the soup to simmer for an

additional 5-10 minutes to let the flavors meld together.

6. **Taste and Adjust:** Taste the soup and adjust the seasoning with more salt and pepper if needed.

7. **Serve:** Ladle the turkey and rice soup into bowls. Garnish with chopped fresh parsley if desired. Serve hot.

Grilled Salmon:

Ingredients:

- 2 salmon filets (6-8 ounces each), skinless and boneless
- 1 tablespoon olive oil
- 1/2 teaspoon salt (or to taste)
- 1/4 teaspoon black pepper (or to taste)
- 1/2 teaspoon dried dill (optional, for flavor)
- 1/2 teaspoon lemon zest (optional, for flavor)

- Lemon wedges for garnish (optional)

Instructions:

1. **Preheat the Grill:** Preheat your grill to medium-high heat. Make sure the grates are clean and lightly oiled to prevent sticking.

2. **Prepare the Salmon:** Rinse the salmon filets under cold water and pat them dry with paper towels. Place them on a clean plate.

3. **Season the Salmon:** Drizzle the olive oil over both sides of the salmon filets. Season the salmon with salt and black pepper. For extra flavor, you can sprinkle dried dill and lemon zest on both sides as well. Gently press the seasonings onto the salmon to ensure they stick.

4. **Grill the Salmon:** Place the salmon filets directly on the preheated grill

grates. Grill for about 4-5 minutes per side, depending on the thickness of the filets. You can use a grill brush or spatula to carefully flip them. Salmon is done when it easily flakes with a fork and has grill marks on both sides.

5. **Rest and Serve:** Once the salmon is cooked, remove it from the grill and let it rest for a few minutes. This allows the juices to redistribute, keeping the fish moist. Serve the grilled salmon with lemon wedges on the side for added flavor, if desired.

6. **Optional Side:** For a gentle side dish, consider serving the grilled salmon with a side of mashed potatoes and steamed, well-cooked vegetables, such as carrots or green beans.

Roasted Vegetables with Quinoa:

Ingredients:

For the Roasted Vegetables:

- 2 cups mixed vegetables (e.g., carrots, zucchini, bell peppers, and tomatoes), cut into bite-sized pieces
- 2 tablespoons olive oil
- 1/2 teaspoon dried thyme
- 1/2 teaspoon dried rosemary
- Salt and pepper to taste

For the Quinoa:

- 1 cup quinoa, rinsed and drained
- 2 cups water or low-sodium vegetable broth
- 1/2 teaspoon salt

Instructions:

Roasted Vegetables:

1. **Preheat the Oven:** Preheat your oven to 400°F (200°C).

2. **Prepare the Vegetables:** In a large mixing bowl, combine the mixed vegetables with olive oil, dried thyme, dried rosemary, salt, and pepper. Toss well to coat the vegetables evenly with the seasonings.

3. **Roast the Vegetables:** Spread the seasoned vegetables in a single layer on a baking sheet lined with parchment paper or a silicone baking mat. Roast in the preheated oven for 20-25 minutes, or until the vegetables are tender and slightly caramelized, stirring them once or twice during cooking.

Quinoa:

1. **Rinse Quinoa:** While the vegetables are roasting, rinse the quinoa under cold

running water in a fine-mesh strainer. This helps remove any bitter taste.

2. **Cook Quinoa:** In a saucepan, combine the rinsed quinoa, water (or vegetable broth), and salt. Bring the mixture to a boil, then reduce the heat to low, cover, and simmer for 15-20 minutes, or until the quinoa is tender and the liquid is absorbed. Fluff the cooked quinoa with a fork.

Assembly:

1. **Serve:** Divide the cooked quinoa among serving plates or bowls. Top with the roasted vegetables.

2. **Optional Additions:** You can add a squeeze of lemon juice or a drizzle of olive oil for extra flavor. Fresh herbs like

parsley or basil also make great garnishes.

Tofu and Vegetable Stir-Fry:

Ingredients:

For the Stir-Fry Sauce:

- 2 tablespoons low-sodium soy sauce
- 1 tablespoon rice vinegar
- 1 tablespoon honey (or a suitable substitute like maple syrup)
- 1 teaspoon cornstarch (optional, for thickening)

For the Stir-Fry:

- 1 block (about 14 ounces) firm or extra-firm tofu, cubed
- 2 tablespoons olive oil or canola oil
- 1 bell pepper, sliced into strips
- 1 small zucchini, sliced
- 1 cup broccoli florets

- 1 cup snap peas, trimmed

- 2 cloves garlic, minced

- 1/2 teaspoon grated fresh ginger

- Salt and pepper to taste

- Cooked white rice or quinoa (optional, for serving)

Instructions:

Stir-Fry Sauce:

1. In a small bowl, whisk together the soy sauce, rice vinegar, honey, and cornstarch (if using). Set aside.

Tofu:

1. To prepare the tofu, press it to remove excess moisture. You can do this by wrapping the tofu block in a clean

kitchen towel and placing something heavy on top, like a cast-iron skillet. Let it sit for 15-20 minutes. Then, cut the tofu into bite-sized cubes.

2. In a large skillet or wok, heat 1 tablespoon of oil over medium-high heat. Add the tofu cubes and stir-fry until they are golden brown and crispy on all sides. This may take about 10-12 minutes. Once done, transfer the tofu to a plate and set it aside.

Stir-Fry:

1. In the same skillet or wok, add the remaining 1 tablespoon of oil. Add the minced garlic and grated ginger, and stir-fry for about 30 seconds, until fragrant.

2. Add the sliced bell pepper, zucchini, broccoli, and snap peas to the skillet.

Stir-fry the vegetables for 5-7 minutes or until they are tender-crisp.

3. Return the crispy tofu to the skillet with the cooked vegetables. Pour the stir-fry sauce over the tofu and vegetables.

4. Toss everything together and cook for an additional 2-3 minutes, or until the sauce has thickened slightly.

5. Season with salt and pepper to taste.

Serve:

Serve your tofu and vegetable stir-fry over cooked white rice or quinoa if desired.

Mashed Sweet Potatoes:

Ingredients:

- 2 large sweet potatoes, peeled and cut into 1-inch chunks

- 2 tablespoons unsalted butter (optional)

- 1/4 cup low-fat milk or lactose-free milk (optional)

- Salt and pepper to taste

- Fresh chopped herbs like chives or parsley (optional, for garnish)

Instructions:

1. **Prepare the Sweet Potatoes:** Peel the sweet potatoes and cut them into 1-inch chunks. This will help them cook more quickly and evenly.

2. **Boil the Sweet Potatoes:** Place the sweet potato chunks in a large pot of water. Bring the water to a boil over high heat, then reduce the heat to medium-low and simmer for about 15-20 minutes or until the sweet potatoes are fork-tender. Be careful not to overcook, as they can become too mushy.

3. **Drain and Mash:** Drain the cooked sweet potatoes in a colander and return them to the pot. Use a potato masher or a fork to mash the sweet potatoes until they are smooth and lump-free.

4. **Add Butter and Milk (Optional):** If you prefer a creamier texture, you can add 2 tablespoons of unsalted butter and 1/4 cup of low-fat milk or lactose-free milk to the mashed sweet potatoes. Gently stir until the butter is melted, and the mixture is well combined. Adjust the amount of milk to achieve your desired consistency.

5. **Season:** Season the mashed sweet potatoes with salt and pepper to taste. Be mindful not to overdo the seasoning, especially if you have dietary restrictions due to diverticulitis.

6. **Garnish (Optional):** For extra flavor and visual appeal, garnish the mashed sweet potatoes with fresh chopped herbs like chives or parsley.

7. **Serve:** Serve the mashed sweet potatoes as a side dish alongside a protein source like baked chicken or grilled fish for a balanced meal.

Baked Turkey Meatballs:

Ingredients:

For the Turkey Meatballs:

- 1 pound lean ground turkey
- 1/2 cup old-fashioned oats (finely ground in a food processor)
- 1/4 cup grated carrot (peeled)
- 1/4 cup grated zucchini
- 1/4 cup finely chopped spinach
- 1/4 cup finely chopped onion

- 1 clove garlic, minced

- 1/2 teaspoon dried oregano

- 1/2 teaspoon dried basil

- Salt and pepper to taste

For the Tomato Sauce:

- 1 can (14 ounces) low-sodium diced tomatoes

- 1 clove garlic, minced

- 1/2 teaspoon dried basil

- Salt and pepper to taste

Instructions:

Turkey Meatballs:

1. **Preheat the Oven:** Preheat your oven to 375°F (190°C). Line a baking sheet with parchment paper or lightly grease it.

2. **Prepare Vegetables:** Grate the carrot and zucchini, finely chop the spinach, and finely chop the onion. You can use a

food processor to make the oats finer as well.

3. **Combine Ingredients:** In a mixing bowl, combine the ground turkey, finely ground oats, grated carrot, grated zucchini, chopped spinach, chopped onion, minced garlic, dried oregano, dried basil, salt, and pepper. Mix well until all the ingredients are evenly incorporated.

4. **Shape Meatballs:** Shape the mixture into meatballs, about 1 to 1.5 inches in diameter. You should be able to make approximately 16 meatballs.

5. **Bake:** Place the meatballs on the prepared baking sheet. Bake in the preheated oven for 20-25 minutes, or until they are cooked through and no longer pink in the center. The internal

temperature of the meatballs should reach 165°F (74°C).

Tomato Sauce:

1. While the meatballs are baking, prepare the tomato sauce. In a small saucepan, combine the diced tomatoes (with their juice), minced garlic, dried basil, salt, and pepper. Heat the sauce over medium-low heat, stirring occasionally, until it's heated through.

2. Once the meatballs are done baking, you can either serve them with the tomato sauce drizzled on top or gently simmer them in the sauce for a few minutes for extra flavor.

Serve:

Serve the baked turkey meatballs with the tomato sauce and your choice of cooked pasta, rice, or steamed vegetables

Creamy Spinach Soup:

Ingredients:

- 4 cups fresh spinach leaves, washed and chopped
- 1 small potato, peeled and diced
- 1 small onion, chopped
- 2 cloves garlic, minced
- 2 cups low-sodium vegetable broth
- 1 cup low-fat milk or lactose-free milk
- 1 tablespoon olive oil
- Salt and pepper to taste
- Pinch of nutmeg (optional, for flavor)

Instructions:

1. **Sauté Vegetables:** In a large pot, heat the olive oil over medium heat. Add the chopped onion and minced garlic. Sauté for 2-3 minutes until they become translucent.

2. **Add Potato:** Add the diced potato to the pot and continue to cook for another 2-3 minutes, stirring occasionally.

3. **Add Spinach:** Stir in the chopped spinach and sauté for an additional 2 minutes until the spinach starts to wilt.

4. **Add Broth:** Pour in the low-sodium vegetable broth. Bring the mixture to a boil, then reduce the heat to a simmer. Cover the pot and let it simmer for about 15-20 minutes, or until the potatoes are tender.

5. **Blend:** Using an immersion blender or a regular blender, carefully blend the soup until it's smooth and creamy. If using a

regular blender, allow the soup to cool slightly before blending, and blend in batches if necessary. Be cautious when blending hot liquids.

6. **Return to Pot:** Return the blended soup to the pot over low heat.

7. **Add Milk:** Stir in the low-fat milk or lactose-free milk to achieve your desired creaminess. Add more or less milk as needed. If you prefer a thicker soup, you can skip or reduce the amount of milk.

8. **Season:** Season the soup with salt, pepper, and a pinch of nutmeg (if desired). Adjust the seasoning to your taste.

9. **Simmer:** Let the soup simmer for an additional 5-10 minutes to allow the flavors to meld together.

10. **Serve:** Ladle the creamy spinach soup into bowls and serve hot. You can

garnish with a sprinkle of fresh chopped parsley or a dollop of low-fat yogurt if desired.

Baked Pork Tenderloin:

Ingredients:

- 1 pork tenderloin (about 1 to 1.5 pounds)
- 1 tablespoon olive oil
- 1/2 teaspoon salt (or to taste)
- 1/4 teaspoon black pepper (or to taste)
- 1/2 teaspoon dried thyme (optional, for flavor)
- 1/2 teaspoon dried rosemary (optional, for flavor)
- 1/2 teaspoon garlic powder (optional, for flavor)
- 1/2 teaspoon paprika (optional, for flavor)

Instructions:

1. **Preheat the Oven:** Preheat your oven to 375°F (190°C).

2. **Prepare the Pork Tenderloin:** Trim any excess fat or silver skin from the pork tenderloin. Pat it dry with paper towels. Place it on a clean plate or cutting board.

3. **Season the Pork:** Drizzle the olive oil over the pork tenderloin. Season it with salt and black pepper. If you want to add more flavor, sprinkle on the dried thyme, dried rosemary, garlic powder, and paprika. Gently rub the seasonings into the pork to coat evenly.

4. **Sear (Optional):** In a large ovenproof skillet, heat a bit of olive oil over medium-high heat. Once hot, sear the pork tenderloin on all sides until it's browned. This step is optional but adds extra flavor and color to the meat.

5. **Bake:** If you didn't sear the pork, place it directly on a baking sheet or in an ovenproof skillet. Bake in the preheated oven for about 20-30 minutes, or until the internal temperature reaches 145°F (63°C) when measured with a meat thermometer. Cooking time may vary depending on the thickness of the tenderloin.

6. **Rest and Serve:** Once cooked, remove the pork from the oven and let it rest for a few minutes before slicing. This allows the juices to redistribute and keeps the pork tender and moist. Slice the pork tenderloin into thin rounds and serve.

7. **Optional Side:** For a gentle side dish, consider serving the baked pork tenderloin with cooked carrots, mashed potatoes, or steamed green beans.

Ingredients:

- 1 cup Arborio rice (risotto rice)
- 2 cups peeled and diced butternut squash
- 1 small onion, finely chopped
- 2 cloves garlic, minced
- 4 cups low-sodium vegetable broth
- 1/2 cup dry white wine (optional, can be omitted if alcohol is a concern)
- 2 tablespoons olive oil
- 1/4 teaspoon dried thyme
- Salt and pepper to taste
- Grated Parmesan cheese for garnish (optional)
- Fresh chopped parsley for garnish (optional)

Instructions:

1. **Prepare the Butternut Squash:** Peel and dice the butternut squash into small, bite-sized pieces. Set aside.

2. **Warm the Broth:** In a separate saucepan, heat the low-sodium vegetable broth over low heat. Keep it warm throughout the cooking process.

3. **Sauté Onion and Garlic:** In a large skillet or wide saucepan, heat the olive oil over medium heat. Add the chopped onion and minced garlic. Sauté for 2-3 minutes until the onion becomes translucent.

4. **Toast the Rice:** Add the Arborio rice to the skillet with the sautéed onion and garlic. Stir to coat the rice with the oil and cook for 1-2 minutes, allowing it to toast slightly.

5. **Deglaze with Wine (Optional):** If using white wine, pour it into the skillet with the rice and stir. Allow it to simmer and reduce until mostly absorbed by the rice.

6. **Add Butternut Squash:** Stir in the diced butternut squash and dried thyme. Season with a pinch of salt and pepper.

7. **Begin Adding Broth:** Start adding the warm vegetable broth one ladle at a time, stirring constantly. Allow the liquid to be absorbed by the rice before adding more. Continue this process, adding broth and stirring, until the rice and butternut squash are tender and creamy. This typically takes about 18-20 minutes.

8. **Finish and Season:** Taste the risotto and adjust the seasoning with salt and pepper as needed. The rice should be creamy and the butternut squash tender.

9. **Serve:** Ladle the butternut squash risotto onto serving plates. If desired, garnish with grated Parmesan cheese and fresh chopped parsley for added flavor and presentation.

Baked Chicken Thighs:

Ingredients:

- 4 boneless, skinless chicken thighs
- 2 tablespoons olive oil
- 1/2 teaspoon dried thyme
- 1/2 teaspoon dried rosemary
- 1/2 teaspoon garlic powder
- Salt and pepper to taste
- 1/2 cup low-sodium chicken broth

Instructions:

1. **Preheat the Oven:** Preheat your oven to 375°F (190°C).

2. **Prepare the Chicken Thighs:** Pat the chicken thighs dry with paper towels and place them in a baking dish.

3. **Season the Chicken:** In a small bowl, combine the olive oil, dried thyme, dried rosemary, garlic powder, salt, and pepper. Mix well to create a seasoning mixture.

4. **Coat the Chicken:** Brush the chicken thighs with the seasoning mixture, making sure to coat them evenly on both sides.

5. **Add Chicken Broth:** Pour the low-sodium chicken broth into the baking dish around the chicken thighs. This helps keep the chicken moist during baking.

6. **Cover and Bake:** Cover the baking dish with aluminum foil to trap in moisture. Bake in the preheated oven for about 30-

35 minutes or until the chicken thighs reach an internal temperature of 165°F (74°C). Cooking time may vary depending on the size and thickness of the thighs.

7. **Rest and Serve:** Once cooked, remove the chicken from the oven and let it rest for a few minutes before serving. This allows the juices to redistribute and keeps the chicken moist.

8. **Serve:** Baked chicken thighs can be served with well-cooked, easily digestible side dishes such as mashed potatoes or steamed carrots.

Salmon and Asparagus Foil Packets:

Ingredients:

- 2 salmon filets (6-8 ounces each), skinless and boneless

- 1 bunch of fresh asparagus spears

- 2 tablespoons olive oil

- 2 cloves garlic, minced

- 1 lemon, thinly sliced

- 1 teaspoon dried dill (or fresh dill if preferred)

- Salt and pepper to taste

Instructions:

1. **Preheat the Oven:** Preheat your oven to 375°F (190°C).

2. **Prepare Foil Packets:** Tear off two large sheets of aluminum foil, each about 12 inches in length. Place one salmon filet in the center of each sheet.

3. **Prepare Asparagus:** Wash and trim the tough ends of the asparagus spears. Divide the asparagus evenly between the two foil packets, arranging them next to the salmon filets.

4. **Season:** Drizzle 1 tablespoon of olive oil over each salmon filet and the asparagus. Sprinkle minced garlic, dried dill, salt, and pepper evenly over the salmon and asparagus.

5. **Lemon Slices:** Place a few thin lemon slices on top of each salmon filet for added flavor and moisture.

6. **Wrap Foil Packets:** Carefully fold the sides of the foil over the salmon and asparagus, creating a packet. Ensure the packet is sealed tightly, so the steam doesn't escape during baking.

7. **Bake:** Place the foil packets on a baking sheet and bake in the preheated oven for approximately 15-20 minutes, or until the salmon flakes easily with a fork and the asparagus is tender. Cooking time may vary depending on the thickness of the salmon.

8. **Serve:** Carefully open the foil packets (watch out for hot steam) and transfer the salmon and asparagus to serving plates. You can drizzle any juices from the packets over the salmon for extra flavor.

Chickpea and Spinach Curry:

Ingredients:

- 1 can (15 ounces) chickpeas, drained and rinsed
- 1 tablespoon olive oil
- 1 small onion, finely chopped
- 2 cloves garlic, minced
- 1-inch piece of fresh ginger, grated
- 1 tablespoon curry powder (adjust to taste)
- 1 teaspoon ground cumin
- 1 teaspoon ground coriander
- 1/2 teaspoon turmeric
- 1/2 teaspoon paprika

- 1 can (14 ounces) diced tomatoes (low-sodium if available)
- 1 can (14 ounces) light coconut milk
- 4 cups fresh spinach leaves, washed and chopped
- Salt and pepper to taste
- Fresh cilantro leaves for garnish (optional)

Instructions:

1. **Heat Oil:** In a large skillet or saucepan, heat the olive oil over medium heat.

2. **Sauté Onion and Garlic:** Add the chopped onion and sauté for 2-3 minutes until it becomes translucent. Stir in the minced garlic and grated ginger, and sauté for an additional 1-2 minutes until fragrant.

3. **Add Spices:** Add the curry powder, ground cumin, ground coriander,

turmeric, and paprika to the skillet. Stir well to coat the onions and spices evenly. Cook for about 1-2 minutes to toast the spices.

4. **Add Tomatoes:** Pour in the diced tomatoes with their juice. Stir to combine, and let the mixture simmer for 5 minutes, allowing the flavors to meld together.

5. **Add Coconut Milk and Chickpeas:** Pour in the light coconut milk and add the drained and rinsed chickpeas. Stir well to combine. Allow the mixture to simmer for another 5-7 minutes, ensuring the chickpeas are heated through.

6. **Add Spinach:** Gently fold in the chopped spinach leaves. Let them wilt and cook for 2-3 minutes, or until the spinach is tender.

7. **Season:** Season the chickpea and spinach curry with salt and pepper to taste. Adjust the seasoning as needed.

8. **Garnish and Serve:** If desired, garnish the curry with fresh cilantro leaves before serving.

9. **Serve:** Serve the chickpea and spinach curry over cooked white rice or quinoa for a complete meal.

CHAPTER 5

SATISFYING STEW AND SOUPS

Stews:

Chicken and Rice Stew:

Ingredients:

- 1 pound boneless, skinless chicken breasts or thighs, cut into bite-sized pieces
- 1 cup white rice (long-grain or basmati)
- 4 cups low-sodium chicken broth
- 2 carrots, peeled and chopped
- 2 celery stalks, chopped
- 1 cup zucchini, chopped
- 1 cup green beans, trimmed and chopped
- 1 cup canned diced tomatoes (without seeds)

- 1/2 teaspoon dried thyme
- 1/2 teaspoon dried rosemary
- Salt and pepper to taste
- 1 tablespoon olive oil
- Fresh parsley for garnish (optional)

Instructions:

1. In a large pot or Dutch oven, heat the olive oil over medium heat.

2. Add the chopped chicken pieces and cook until they are no longer pink, about 5-7 minutes. Remove the chicken from the pot and set it aside.

3. In the same pot, add the chopped carrots, celery, zucchini, and green beans. Sauté the vegetables for about 5 minutes until they start to soften.

4. Stir in the dried thyme and rosemary, and season with a pinch of salt and pepper.

5. Add the canned diced tomatoes (make sure they don't contain seeds) and cook for another 2-3 minutes.

6. Return the cooked chicken to the pot.

7. Add the white rice to the pot and stir everything together.

8. Pour in the chicken broth and bring the mixture to a boil.

9. Reduce the heat to low, cover the pot, and let it simmer for about 20-25 minutes, or until the rice is tender and the chicken is fully cooked.

10. Taste the stew and adjust the seasoning with more salt and pepper if needed.

11. Serve the chicken and rice stew hot, garnished with fresh parsley if desired.

Turkey and Vegetable Stew:

Ingredients:

- 1 pound lean ground turkey
- 4 cups low-sodium chicken or turkey broth
- 1 cup carrots, peeled and chopped
- 1 cup celery, chopped
- 1 cup zucchini, chopped
- 1 cup green beans, trimmed and chopped
- 1 cup canned diced tomatoes (without seeds)
- 1/2 cup quinoa or white rice
- 1/2 teaspoon dried thyme
- 1/2 teaspoon dried rosemary
- Salt and pepper to taste
- 1 tablespoon olive oil
- Fresh parsley for garnish (optional)

Instructions:

1. In a large pot or Dutch oven, heat the olive oil over medium heat.

2. Add the ground turkey and cook until it's no longer pink, breaking it apart into small pieces with a spoon. This should take about 5-7 minutes. Remove the cooked turkey from the pot and set it aside.

3. In the same pot, add the chopped carrots, celery, zucchini, and green beans. Sauté the vegetables for about 5 minutes until they begin to soften.

4. Stir in the dried thyme and rosemary, and season with a pinch of salt and pepper.

5. Add the canned diced tomatoes (ensure they do not contain seeds) and cook for an additional 2-3 minutes.

6. Return the cooked turkey to the pot.

7. Add the quinoa or white rice to the pot and mix everything together.

8. Pour in the chicken or turkey broth and bring the mixture to a boil.

9. Reduce the heat to low, cover the pot, and let it simmer for about 15-20 minutes, or until the quinoa or rice is fully cooked and the vegetables are tender.

10. Taste the stew and adjust the seasoning with more salt and pepper if needed.

11. Serve the turkey and vegetable stew hot, garnished with fresh parsley if desired.

Lentil and Carrot Stew:

Ingredients:

- 1 cup dried green or brown lentils, rinsed and drained
- 4 cups low-sodium vegetable broth
- 2 cups carrots, peeled and chopped
- 1 cup celery, chopped
- 1 cup onion, finely chopped

- 2 cloves garlic, minced

- 1 teaspoon ground cumin

- 1/2 teaspoon ground coriander

- 1/2 teaspoon dried thyme

- Salt and pepper to taste

- 2 tablespoons olive oil

- Fresh parsley for garnish (optional)

Instructions:

1. In a large pot or Dutch oven, heat the olive oil over medium heat.

2. Add the chopped onions and garlic. Sauté for about 2-3 minutes until they become fragrant and translucent.

3. Stir in the ground cumin, ground coriander, and dried thyme. Cook for an additional minute to toast the spices.

4. Add the chopped carrots and celery to the pot. Sauté for another 5 minutes until they begin to soften.

5. Pour in the rinsed lentils and vegetable broth. Bring the mixture to a boil.

6. Reduce the heat to low, cover the pot, and let it simmer for about 25-30 minutes, or until the lentils and vegetables are tender.

7. Season the stew with salt and pepper to taste. Adjust the seasoning as needed.

8. Serve the lentil and carrot stew hot, garnished with fresh parsley if desired.

Sweet Potato and Turkey Stew:

Ingredients:

- 1 pound lean ground turkey
- 2 medium sweet potatoes, peeled and chopped into small cubes
- 4 cups low-sodium chicken or turkey broth
- 1 cup carrots, peeled and chopped
- 1 cup celery, chopped

- 1 cup onion, finely chopped
- 2 cloves garlic, minced
- 1 teaspoon dried thyme
- 1/2 teaspoon dried rosemary
- Salt and pepper to taste
- 2 tablespoons olive oil
- Fresh parsley for garnish (optional)

Instructions:

1. In a large pot or Dutch oven, heat the olive oil over medium heat.

2. Add the chopped onions and garlic. Sauté for about 2-3 minutes until they become fragrant and translucent.

3. Add the ground turkey and cook until it's no longer pink, breaking it apart into small pieces with a spoon. This should take about 5-7 minutes. Remove the cooked turkey from the pot and set it aside.

4. In the same pot, add the chopped sweet potatoes, carrots, and celery. Sauté the vegetables for about 5 minutes until they begin to soften.

5. Stir in the dried thyme and dried rosemary, and season with a pinch of salt and pepper.

6. Return the cooked turkey to the pot.

7. Pour in the chicken or turkey broth and bring the mixture to a boil.

8. Reduce the heat to low, cover the pot, and let it simmer for about 15-20 minutes, or until the sweet potatoes are tender and the flavors meld together.

9. Taste the stew and adjust the seasoning with more salt and pepper if needed.

10. Serve the sweet potato and turkey stew hot, garnished with fresh parsley if desired.

Zucchini and Tomato Stew:

Ingredients:

- 2 medium zucchinis, chopped
- 2 cups canned diced tomatoes (without seeds)
- 1 cup low-sodium vegetable broth
- 1 cup carrots, peeled and chopped
- 1 cup celery, chopped
- 1 cup onion, finely chopped
- 2 cloves garlic, minced
- 1 teaspoon dried basil
- 1/2 teaspoon dried oregano
- Salt and pepper to taste
- 2 tablespoons olive oil
- Fresh basil leaves for garnish (optional)

Instructions:

1. In a large pot or Dutch oven, heat the olive oil over medium heat.

2. Add the chopped onions and garlic. Sauté for about 2-3 minutes until they become fragrant and translucent.

3. Add the chopped carrots and celery to the pot. Sauté for another 5 minutes until they begin to soften.

4. Stir in the dried basil and dried oregano, and season with a pinch of salt and pepper.

5. Add the chopped zucchinis to the pot and sauté for an additional 3-4 minutes.

6. Pour in the canned diced tomatoes (ensure they do not contain seeds) and vegetable broth. Bring the mixture to a boil.

7. Reduce the heat to low, cover the pot, and let it simmer for about 15-20 minutes, or until the vegetables are tender and the flavors meld together.

8. Taste the stew and adjust the seasoning with more salt and pepper if needed.

9. Serve the zucchini and tomato stew hot, garnished with fresh basil leaves if desired.

Spinach and Potato Soup:

Ingredients:

- 2 large russet potatoes, peeled and diced
- 4 cups low-sodium vegetable broth
- 4 cups fresh spinach, chopped
- 1 cup onion, finely chopped
- 2 cloves garlic, minced
- 1/2 cup celery, chopped
- 1/2 cup leeks, chopped (optional)
- 1/2 teaspoon dried thyme
- Salt and pepper to taste
- 2 tablespoons olive oil

- Plain Greek yogurt or sour cream for garnish (optional)

Instructions:

1. In a large pot, heat the olive oil over medium heat.
2. Add the chopped onions and garlic. Sauté for about 2-3 minutes until they become fragrant and translucent.
3. If using leeks, add them to the pot along with the celery. Sauté for an additional 5 minutes until they begin to soften.
4. Stir in the dried thyme and season with a pinch of salt and pepper.
5. Add the diced potatoes to the pot and sauté for another 2-3 minutes.
6. Pour in the vegetable broth and bring the mixture to a boil.

7. Reduce the heat to low, cover the pot, and let it simmer for about 15-20 minutes, or until the potatoes are tender.

8. Once the potatoes are soft, use an immersion blender or a regular blender to carefully puree the soup until it's smooth and creamy.

9. Return the soup to the pot and add the chopped spinach. Simmer for an additional 5 minutes, or until the spinach wilts and is tender.

10. Taste the soup and adjust the seasoning with more salt and pepper if needed.

11. Serve the spinach and potato soup hot, garnished with a dollop of plain Greek yogurt or sour cream if desired.

Broccoli and Cheddar Soup:

Ingredients:

- 4 cups fresh broccoli florets, chopped
- 2 cups low-sodium vegetable broth
- 1 cup sharp cheddar cheese, grated
- 1 cup onion, finely chopped
- 2 cloves garlic, minced
- 1/2 cup celery, chopped
- 2 tablespoons unsalted butter
- 2 tablespoons all-purpose flour
- 2 cups low-fat milk (or a lactose-free alternative)
- Salt and pepper to taste
- Dash of nutmeg (optional)
- Chopped chives or green onions for garnish (optional)

Instructions:

1. In a large pot, melt the unsalted butter over medium heat.

2. Add the chopped onions, garlic, and celery. Sauté for about 2-3 minutes until they become fragrant and translucent.

3. Stir in the all-purpose flour to create a roux. Cook for an additional 2-3 minutes, stirring constantly until the mixture is lightly golden.

4. Slowly pour in the low-fat milk while whisking continuously to avoid lumps. Continue to whisk until the mixture thickens, usually within 5-7 minutes.

5. Add the low-sodium vegetable broth and chopped broccoli to the pot. Bring the mixture to a boil, then reduce the heat to low, cover the pot, and let it simmer for about 15-20 minutes, or until the broccoli is tender.

6. Using an immersion blender or a regular blender (in batches), carefully puree the

soup until it's smooth and creamy. Be cautious when blending hot liquids.

7. Return the soup to the pot and stir in the grated cheddar cheese until it's fully melted and the soup is creamy.

8. Season the soup with salt, pepper, and a dash of nutmeg if desired. Adjust the seasoning to taste.

9. Serve the broccoli and cheddar soup hot, garnished with chopped chives or green onions if desired.

Carrot Ginger Soup:

Ingredients:

- 1 pound carrots, peeled and chopped
- 1 medium potato, peeled and chopped
- 1 onion, chopped
- 2 cloves garlic, minced
- 2 tablespoons fresh ginger, minced

- 4 cups low-sodium vegetable broth

- 2 tablespoons olive oil

- Salt and pepper to taste

- Fresh cilantro or chives for garnish (optional)

Instructions:

1. In a large pot, heat the olive oil over medium heat.

2. Add the chopped onions and garlic. Sauté for about 2-3 minutes until they become fragrant and translucent.

3. Stir in the minced ginger and continue to sauté for an additional minute.

4. Add the chopped carrots and potato to the pot. Sauté for another 5 minutes, allowing them to soften slightly.

5. Pour in the low-sodium vegetable broth and bring the mixture to a boil.

6. Reduce the heat to low, cover the pot, and let it simmer for about 20-25 minutes, or until the carrots and potato are tender.

7. Use an immersion blender or a regular blender (in batches, if necessary) to puree the soup until it's smooth and creamy. Be cautious when blending hot liquids.

8. Return the soup to the pot and season with salt and pepper to taste. Adjust the seasoning as needed.

9. Heat the soup for an additional 5 minutes on low heat, stirring occasionally.

10. Serve the carrot ginger soup hot, garnished with fresh cilantro or chives if desired.

Red Lentil Soup:

Ingredients:

- 1 cup dried red lentils, rinsed and drained
- 4 cups low-sodium vegetable broth
- 1 cup carrots, peeled and chopped
- 1 cup celery, chopped
- 1 cup onion, finely chopped
- 2 cloves garlic, minced
- 1 teaspoon ground cumin
- 1/2 teaspoon ground coriander
- Salt and pepper to taste
- 2 tablespoons olive oil
- Fresh cilantro or parsley for garnish (optional)
- Lemon wedges for serving (optional)

Instructions:

1. In a large pot, heat the olive oil over medium heat.

2. Add the chopped onions and garlic. Sauté for about 2-3 minutes until they become fragrant and translucent.

3. Stir in the ground cumin and ground coriander. Cook for an additional minute to toast the spices.

4. Add the chopped carrots and celery to the pot. Sauté for another 5 minutes until they begin to soften.

5. Pour in the rinsed red lentils and vegetable broth. Bring the mixture to a boil.

6. Reduce the heat to low, cover the pot, and let it simmer for about 20-25 minutes, or until the lentils are tender and the flavors meld together.

7. Using an immersion blender or a regular blender (in batches, if necessary), carefully puree the soup until it's smooth

and creamy. Be cautious when blending hot liquids.

8. Return the soup to the pot and heat it for an additional 5 minutes on low heat.

9. Season the soup with salt and pepper to taste. Adjust the seasoning as needed.

10. Serve the red lentil soup hot, garnished with fresh cilantro or parsley if desired. Squeezing a little lemon juice over each bowl of soup can add a refreshing twist.

Pea and Mint Soup:

Ingredients:

- 2 cups frozen peas
- 4 cups low-sodium vegetable broth
- 1 cup onion, finely chopped
- 1 cup celery, chopped
- 2 cloves garlic, minced
- 1/2 cup fresh mint leaves, chopped

- Salt and pepper to taste

- 2 tablespoons olive oil

- Greek yogurt or sour cream for garnish (optional)

- Fresh mint leaves for garnish (optional)

Instructions:

1. In a large pot, heat the olive oil over medium heat.

2. Add the chopped onions and garlic. Sauté for about 2-3 minutes until they become fragrant and translucent.

3. Add the chopped celery to the pot and sauté for another 5 minutes until it begins to soften.

4. Stir in the frozen peas and chopped mint leaves. Sauté for an additional 2-3 minutes.

5. Pour in the low-sodium vegetable broth and bring the mixture to a boil.

6. Reduce the heat to low, cover the pot, and let it simmer for about 10-15 minutes, or until the peas are tender.

7. Using an immersion blender or a regular blender (in batches, if necessary), carefully puree the soup until it's smooth and creamy. Be cautious when blending hot liquids.

8. Return the soup to the pot and heat it for an additional 5 minutes on low heat.

9. Season the soup with salt and pepper to taste. Adjust the seasoning as needed.

10. Serve the pea and mint soup hot, garnished with a dollop of Greek yogurt or sour cream and a few fresh mint leaves if desired.

Minestrone Soup:

Ingredients:

- 1 cup whole grain pasta (choose a type that is easy on your digestion, such as small shells or penne)
- 4 cups low-sodium vegetable broth
- 1 cup canned diced tomatoes (without seeds)
- 1 cup zucchini, chopped
- 1 cup carrots, peeled and chopped
- 1 cup celery, chopped
- 1 cup green beans, trimmed and chopped
- 1 cup canned kidney beans, drained and rinsed
- 1 cup canned cannellini beans, drained and rinsed
- 1 cup spinach or kale, chopped
- 1 cup onion, finely chopped
- 2 cloves garlic, minced
- 1 teaspoon dried basil
- 1/2 teaspoon dried oregano
- Salt and pepper to taste

- 2 tablespoons olive oil

- Grated Parmesan cheese for garnish (optional)

- Fresh basil leaves for garnish (optional)

Instructions:

1. In a large pot, heat the olive oil over medium heat.

2. Add the chopped onions and garlic. Sauté for about 2-3 minutes until they become fragrant and translucent.

3. Stir in the dried basil and dried oregano. Cook for an additional minute to release the flavors.

4. Add the chopped carrots, celery, and zucchini to the pot. Sauté for about 5 minutes until they begin to soften.

5. Pour in the low-sodium vegetable broth and bring the mixture to a boil.

6. Add the diced tomatoes, green beans, and pasta to the pot. Reduce the heat to low, cover the pot, and let it simmer for about 10-12 minutes, or until the pasta is al dente.

7. Stir in the canned kidney beans, canned cannellini beans, and chopped spinach or kale. Simmer for an additional 2-3 minutes, until the beans are heated through and the greens wilt.

8. Season the soup with salt and pepper to taste. Adjust the seasoning as needed.

9. Serve the Minestrone soup hot, garnished with grated Parmesan cheese and fresh basil leaves if desired.

CHAPTER 6

SIDE DISHES AND SNACKS

Side Dishes:

Steamed Asparagus:

Ingredients:

- 1 bunch of fresh asparagus spears
- 1 tablespoon olive oil
- 1 clove garlic, minced (optional)
- Salt and pepper to taste
- Lemon zest (optional, for added flavor)

Instructions:

1. **Prepare the Asparagus:**

- Start by washing the asparagus thoroughly under cold running water to remove any dirt or sand.

- Trim the tough ends of the asparagus spears. You can do this by holding each spear at both ends and gently bending it until it snaps. The spear will naturally break where the tough part ends.

2. **Steam the Asparagus:**

- Fill a large pot with about 2 inches of water and place a steamer basket inside.

- Bring the water to a boil over medium-high heat.

- Place the trimmed asparagus spears in the steamer basket, making sure they are in a single layer for even cooking.

- Cover the pot with a lid and steam the asparagus for 3-5 minutes, depending on the thickness of the spears. They should become tender but still have a slight crispness. Be careful not to overcook, as overcooking can make them mushy and harder to digest.

3. **Season the Asparagus:**

- While the asparagus is steaming, you can prepare a simple seasoning. In a small saucepan, heat the olive oil over low heat.

- If you like, add minced garlic to the oil and sauté for about 1-2 minutes, just until it becomes fragrant. Be careful not to brown the garlic, as this can make it more irritating for someone with diverticulitis.

- Once the asparagus is done steaming, transfer it to a serving plate.

- Drizzle the garlic-infused olive oil over the asparagus, and season with salt, pepper, and lemon zest (if using). The lemon zest can add a nice, fresh flavor to the dish.

4. **Serve:** Serve the steamed asparagus immediately while it's still warm.

Mashed Butternut Squash:

Ingredients:

- medium-sized butternut squash
- 1-2 tablespoons of olive oil
- Salt and pepper to taste
- A pinch of ground cinnamon (optional, for added flavor)

Instructions:

1. **Prepare the Butternut Squash:** Start by peeling the butternut squash with a vegetable peeler to remove the tough outer skin. Cut it in half lengthwise and scoop out the seeds and pulp using a spoon.

2. **Steam the Butternut Squash:**

- Cut the peeled and seeded butternut squash into chunks or cubes, ensuring they are of relatively uniform size. This will help them cook evenly.

- Place the squash pieces in a steamer basket over a pot of boiling water or use a microwave-safe steaming dish. Steam the squash for about 15-20 minutes or until they become fork-tender. Steaming is a gentle cooking method that preserves the nutrients and is easier on the digestive system compared to boiling.

3. **Mash the Squash:**

- Once the butternut squash is tender, transfer it to a mixing bowl.

- Use a potato masher or a fork to mash the squash until you achieve your desired level of smoothness. Some people prefer a slightly chunky texture, while others like it completely smooth.

4. **Season the Mashed Squash:**

- Drizzle the olive oil over the mashed butternut squash.

- Season with a pinch of salt and pepper to taste. You can start with a small amount and adjust to your preference.

- For added flavor, you can sprinkle a pinch of ground cinnamon over the squash. Cinnamon pairs nicely with the natural sweetness of butternut squash.

5. **Serve:** Transfer the seasoned mashed butternut squash to a serving dish and serve it warm.

Cucumber Salad:

Ingredients:

- 2 medium-sized cucumbers, thinly sliced
- 1/2 red onion, thinly sliced
- 1/4 cup fresh dill, chopped

- 1/4 cup plain yogurt (low-fat or dairy-free alternatives are fine)

- 1 tablespoon extra-virgin olive oil

- 1 tablespoon white wine vinegar or apple cider vinegar

- Salt and pepper to taste

Instructions:

1. **Prepare the Cucumbers:**

- Start by washing and scrubbing the cucumbers thoroughly under cold running water. You can choose to peel them or leave the skin on, depending on your preference. Peeling may be gentler on the digestive system.

- Slice the cucumbers thinly. If you have a mandoline slicer, it can be helpful for achieving consistent thickness.

2. **Slice the Red Onion:** Thinly slice the red onion. If you find raw onion to be too

harsh on your stomach, you can soak the sliced onion in cold water for about 10 minutes to mellow its flavor. Then, drain and pat it dry before using.

3. **Chop the Fresh Dill:** Chop the fresh dill finely. Dill adds a wonderful fresh flavor to the salad.

4. **Prepare the Dressing:**

- In a small bowl, combine the plain yogurt, extra-virgin olive oil, and white wine vinegar. Whisk the dressing until it's well combined.

- Season the dressing with a pinch of salt and pepper. Adjust the seasoning to your taste.

5. **Combine and Toss:** In a large mixing bowl, combine the sliced cucumbers, red onion, and chopped dill.

6. **Add the Dressing:** Pour the yogurt-based dressing over the cucumber mixture.

7. **Toss and Coat:** Gently toss the salad ingredients together to ensure the cucumbers and onions are evenly coated with the dressing.

8. **Chill and Serve:**

- Cover the bowl with plastic wrap or a lid and refrigerate the cucumber salad for at least 30 minutes before serving. Chilling helps the flavors meld together.

- Serve the cucumber salad cold as a refreshing side dish.

Roasted Brussels Sprouts:

Ingredients:

- 1 pound Brussels sprouts
- 2 tablespoons olive oil

- 1/2 teaspoon salt (or to taste)
- 1/4 teaspoon black pepper (or to taste)
- 1/4 teaspoon garlic powder (optional)
- 1/4 teaspoon onion powder (optional)

Instructions:

1. **Preheat the Oven:** Preheat your oven to 425°F (220°C).

2. **Prepare Brussels Sprouts:** Wash the Brussels sprouts thoroughly and trim the tough ends. If any sprouts are significantly larger than the others, cut them in half so that they cook evenly.

3. **Season:** Place the prepared Brussels sprouts in a large bowl. Drizzle the olive oil over them and sprinkle with salt, pepper, garlic powder, and onion powder (if using). Toss the sprouts to ensure they are evenly coated with the oil and seasonings.

4. **Arrange on Baking Sheet:** Line a baking sheet with parchment paper or lightly grease it. Spread the seasoned Brussels sprouts out in a single layer on the baking sheet. Make sure there's some space between each sprout for even roasting.

5. **Roast:** Place the baking sheet in the preheated oven and roast for about 20-25 minutes or until the Brussels sprouts are tender and browned, stirring or shaking the pan occasionally for even cooking.

6. **Serve:** Once the Brussels sprouts are roasted to your liking, remove them from the oven. Allow them to cool for a few minutes before serving.

Baked Sweet Potato Fries:

Ingredients:

- 2 large sweet potatoes

- 2 tablespoons olive oil

- 1/2 teaspoon paprika

- 1/2 teaspoon garlic powder

- 1/2 teaspoon onion powder

- Salt and pepper to taste

- Fresh parsley (optional, for garnish)

Instructions:

1. **Preheat the Oven:** Preheat your oven to 425°F (220°C) and line a baking sheet with parchment paper.

2. **Prepare the Sweet Potatoes:** Wash and peel the sweet potatoes. Cut them into thin strips or fries, ensuring they are of uniform thickness. This helps them cook evenly.

3. **Season the Fries:** In a large mixing bowl, combine the sweet potato strips with olive oil, paprika, garlic powder, and onion powder. Toss the sweet potato

strips until they are evenly coated with the seasoning. Add salt and pepper to taste.

4. **Arrange on Baking Sheet:** Spread the seasoned sweet potato fries in a single layer on the prepared baking sheet. Make sure they are not crowded to allow for even cooking.

5. **Bake:** Place the baking sheet in the preheated oven and bake for about 20-25 minutes, flipping the fries halfway through, or until they are crisp on the outside and tender on the inside. Cooking times may vary, so keep an eye on them.

6. **Garnish and Serve:** Once the sweet potato fries are done, remove them from the oven and let them cool slightly. If desired, garnish with fresh parsley for added flavor and presentation.

7. **Enjoy:** Serve your diverticulitis-friendly baked sweet potato fries as a delicious and nutritious side dish or snack.

Sauteed Spinach:

Ingredients:

- 1 bunch fresh spinach (about 8-10 ounces)
- 2 cloves garlic, minced
- 1 tablespoon olive oil
- Salt and pepper to taste
- Lemon juice (optional, for a touch of acidity)

Instructions:

1. **Wash the Spinach:** Start by washing the fresh spinach thoroughly under running water to remove any dirt or debris. You can also use pre-washed and bagged spinach for convenience.

2. **Prepare the Spinach:** Trim any tough stems from the spinach leaves if needed. You can leave the tender stems on as they are edible.

3. **Heat the Olive Oil:** In a large skillet or frying pan, heat the olive oil over medium heat.

4. **Saute the Garlic:** Add the minced garlic to the heated olive oil and sauté for about 30 seconds, or until it becomes fragrant. Be careful not to let it brown or burn.

5. **Add the Spinach:** Gradually add the washed and prepared spinach to the skillet. You may need to add it in batches if your skillet is not large enough to hold it all at once.

6. **Saute the Spinach:** Using tongs or a spatula, gently toss the spinach in the pan to coat it with the garlic-infused oil.

Continue to sauté for 2-3 minutes or until the spinach begins to wilt.

7. **Season and Finish:** Season the sautéed spinach with salt and pepper to taste. If you like a touch of acidity, you can drizzle some fresh lemon juice over the spinach at this point.

8. **Serve:** Transfer the sautéed spinach to a serving dish and serve it immediately while it's still hot.

Snacks:

Yogurt with Berries:

Ingredients:

- 1 cup plain, low-fat yogurt (Greek or regular)
- 1/2 cup mixed berries (e.g., blueberries, strawberries, raspberries)

- 1 tablespoon honey (optional, for sweetness)

- 1/4 cup chopped nuts (e.g., almonds, walnuts) (optional, for added texture and flavor)

Instructions:

1. **Prepare the Berries:** Wash the mixed berries thoroughly and pat them dry with a paper towel. You can use fresh or frozen berries for this recipe.

2. **Choose the Yogurt:** Select plain, low-fat yogurt as it is typically easier on the digestive system. You can use regular yogurt or Greek yogurt based on your preference.

3. **Assemble the Yogurt:** Scoop the yogurt into a serving bowl.

4. **Add the Berries:** Gently layer the washed berries on top of the yogurt.

5. **Sweeten (Optional):** If you prefer your yogurt with a touch of sweetness, drizzle honey over the berries. Adjust the amount of honey to suit your taste.

6. **Add Nuts (Optional):** For added texture and flavor, sprinkle chopped nuts over the top. Nuts can provide a healthy crunch and are rich in nutrients.

7. **Serve:** Your diverticulitis-friendly Yogurt with Berries is ready to be served. Enjoy it as a nutritious and soothing breakfast or snack.

Banana with Almond Butter:

Ingredients:

- 1 ripe banana
- 1-2 tablespoons almond butter (unsweetened and without added oils)
- 1 teaspoon honey (optional, for sweetness)

- A pinch of cinnamon (optional, for flavor)

Instructions:

1. **Prepare the Banana:** Start by peeling the ripe banana and slicing it into bite-sized rounds or lengthwise halves, depending on your preference.

2. **Choose Almond Butter:** Ensure you select almond butter that is unsweetened and doesn't contain added oils. This helps in keeping it gentle on the digestive system.

3. **Spread the Almond Butter:** Using a butter knife or a spoon, spread a thin layer of almond butter onto each banana slice. Adjust the amount of almond butter to your liking.

4. **Sweeten (Optional):** If you desire a touch of sweetness, drizzle a small

amount of honey over the banana and almond butter. Make sure to add honey according to your taste preferences.

5. **Add Cinnamon (Optional):** For extra flavor, sprinkle a pinch of cinnamon over the top. Cinnamon not only adds a pleasant taste but also offers potential health benefits.

6. **Serve:** Your diverticulitis-friendly Banana with Almond Butter is ready to be enjoyed. This simple and nutritious snack or dessert is packed with fiber, healthy fats, and natural sweetness.

Carrot Sticks with Hummus:

Ingredients:

- Fresh carrots, washed and peeled
- Hummus (store-bought or homemade)
- Fresh parsley (optional, for garnish)
- Paprika (optional, for seasoning)

Instructions:

1. **Prepare the Carrot Sticks:** Wash and peel fresh carrots. Cut them into manageable sticks or strips. Ensure the carrot sticks are of a size that's easy to dip into the hummus.

2. **Choose Hummus:** Opt for plain, low-fat hummus without added spices or ingredients that may trigger diverticulitis symptoms. You can use store-bought hummus or make your own.

3. **Transfer Hummus:** Scoop the desired amount of hummus into a serving bowl.

4. **Garnish (Optional):** If you wish to add some visual appeal and flavor, you can garnish the hummus with a sprinkle of paprika or chopped fresh parsley.

5. **Serve:** Arrange the carrot sticks around the hummus bowl, creating a visually

appealing and diverticulitis-friendly snack or appetizer.

6. **Enjoy:** Dip the carrot sticks into the hummus and enjoy this healthy and nutritious treat. The carrots provide fiber and nutrients, while the hummus offers protein and a creamy texture.

Rice Cakes with Cottage Cheese:

Ingredients:

- 2 rice cakes (choose plain, unsalted, and unflavored rice cakes)
- 1/2 cup low-fat cottage cheese
- 1/2 teaspoon honey (optional, for a touch of sweetness)
- Fresh fruit slices (e.g., strawberries, banana) for topping (optional)

Instructions:

1. **Select Rice Cakes:** Choose plain rice cakes without added salt or flavorings. These are easier on the digestive system.

2. **Spread Cottage Cheese:** Take the rice cakes and spread a generous layer of low-fat cottage cheese on top of each rice cake. Adjust the amount to your preference.

3.

4. **Sweeten (Optional):** If you desire a hint of sweetness, drizzle a small amount of honey over the cottage cheese. This step is entirely optional and can be adjusted based on your taste.

5. **Add Fruit (Optional):** For added flavor and nutrition, consider topping the rice cakes and cottage cheese with fresh fruit slices. Sliced strawberries, bananas, or berries work well.

6. **Serve:** Your diverticulitis-friendly Rice Cakes with Cottage Cheese are now ready to be enjoyed.

7. **Enjoy:** Eat them as a quick and nutritious snack or a light breakfast. This combination provides a balance of protein, carbohydrates, and fiber.

Mixed Nuts:

Ingredients:

- 1/4 cup almonds (unsalted)
- 1/4 cup walnuts (unsalted)
- 1/4 cup peanuts (unsalted)
- 1/4 cup cashews (unsalted)
- 1/4 cup pecans (unsalted)
- 1/4 cup hazelnuts (unsalted)
- 1/4 teaspoon sea salt (optional, for seasoning)

Instructions:

1. **Select and Prepare Nuts:** Choose a variety of unsalted nuts such as almonds, walnuts, peanuts, cashews, pecans, and hazelnuts. Ensure they are whole and not coated in any sugary or spicy seasonings.

2. **Chop or Grind:** To make these nuts diverticulitis-friendly, you'll need to chop or grind them into smaller pieces. You can use a food processor or a knife to achieve the desired consistency. Aim for small, bite-sized pieces.

3. **Optional Seasoning:** If you prefer a bit of seasoning, you can lightly season the mixed nuts with a pinch of sea salt. However, this step is entirely optional and should be done sparingly, especially if you have dietary restrictions related to salt.

4. **Mix Well:** In a bowl, combine the chopped or ground nuts. Toss them gently to ensure an even distribution of different nut varieties.

5. **Store:** Store your diverticulitis-friendly mixed nuts in an airtight container. Keep them in a cool, dry place.

6. **Enjoy in Moderation:** Enjoy your mixed nuts as a healthy, protein-rich snack in moderation. Remember to chew them thoroughly to aid digestion.

Baked Apple Slices:

Ingredients:

- 2 apples (choose a variety that you prefer)
- 1 teaspoon ground cinnamon
- 1/2 teaspoon nutmeg (optional)
- 1-2 teaspoons honey (optional, for sweetness)

- 1 tablespoon lemon juice

- Cooking spray or a light coating of vegetable oil

Instructions:

1. **Preheat the Oven:** Preheat your oven to 350°F (175°C) and line a baking sheet with parchment paper or lightly grease it with cooking spray or vegetable oil.

2. **Prepare the Apples:** Wash the apples thoroughly and remove the cores. You can peel the apples if you prefer, but leaving the skin on adds extra fiber and nutrients.

3. **Slice the Apples:** Slice the apples into thin rounds or wedges, about 1/4 inch thick. You can use an apple slicer for even slices.

4. **Toss with Lemon Juice:** In a mixing bowl, toss the apple slices with lemon

juice. This helps prevent browning and adds a subtle tangy flavor.

5. **Season:** In a separate bowl, combine the ground cinnamon and nutmeg (if using). Sprinkle this mixture evenly over the apple slices. If you'd like to add sweetness, drizzle honey over the apple slices. Toss the apples to ensure even coating.

6. **Arrange on Baking Sheet:** Lay the seasoned apple slices in a single layer on the prepared baking sheet.

7. **Bake:** Place the baking sheet in the preheated oven and bake for about 20-25 minutes or until the apples are tender and slightly caramelized.

8. **Cool and Serve:** Allow the baked apple slices to cool for a few minutes before serving. They can be enjoyed warm or at room temperature.

9. **Enjoy:** Serve these diverticulitis-friendly Baked Apple Slices as a healthy and delicious dessert or snack.

Celery and Peanut Butter:

Ingredients:

- 2-3 celery stalks, washed and trimmed
- 2-3 tablespoons natural peanut butter (unsweetened and without added oils)
- Raisins or dried cranberries (optional, for added sweetness)

Instructions:

1. **Prepare the Celery:** Start by washing the celery stalks thoroughly and trimming the ends. You can leave them whole or cut them into smaller, manageable pieces, depending on your preference.

2. **Choose Peanut Butter:** Opt for natural peanut butter that is unsweetened and doesn't contain added oils. This type of peanut butter is typically smoother and easier to spread.

3. **Spread the Peanut Butter:** Using a butter knife or a spoon, spread a thin layer of natural peanut butter onto the celery stalks. Adjust the amount of peanut butter to your liking.

4. **Add Raisins or Cranberries (Optional):** For a touch of sweetness and extra flavor, consider adding a few raisins or dried cranberries on top of the peanut butter. This step is entirely optional and can be customized to your taste.

5. **Serve:** Arrange the peanut butter-filled celery sticks on a plate or platter,

creating a visually appealing and diverticulitis-friendly snack.

6. **Enjoy:** Dip the celery sticks into the peanut butter and savor this nutritious and satisfying treat.

Rice Cakes with Avocado:

Ingredients:

- 2 rice cakes (choose plain, unsalted, and unflavored rice cakes)
- 1 ripe avocado
- 1/2 lemon (juiced)
- Salt and pepper to taste
- Red pepper flakes (optional, for added flavor and heat)
- Fresh cilantro or parsley leaves (optional, for garnish)

Instructions:

1. **Select Rice Cakes:** Choose plain rice cakes without added salt or flavorings. These are easier on the digestive system.

2. **Prepare Avocado:** Cut the ripe avocado in half, remove the pit, and scoop out the flesh into a bowl.

3. **Mash Avocado:** Mash the avocado with a fork or potato masher until you achieve your desired level of creaminess. You can leave it slightly chunky or make it smooth.

4. **Add Lemon Juice:** Squeeze the juice from half a lemon over the mashed avocado. The lemon juice adds a refreshing citrus flavor and helps prevent the avocado from browning.

5. **Season:** Season the avocado mixture with a pinch of salt and pepper to taste. If you enjoy some heat, you can also sprinkle red pepper flakes.

6. **Spread on Rice Cakes:** Take the plain rice cakes and spread a generous layer of the seasoned mashed avocado on top of each rice cake. Adjust the amount of avocado to your liking.

7. **Garnish (Optional):** If desired, garnish the avocado-topped rice cakes with fresh cilantro or parsley leaves for added flavor and presentation.

8. **Serve:** Your diverticulitis-friendly Rice Cakes with Avocado are now ready to be enjoyed.

9. **Enjoy:** Eat them as a light and nutritious snack or a quick breakfast. This combination provides healthy fats, fiber, and a burst of flavor.

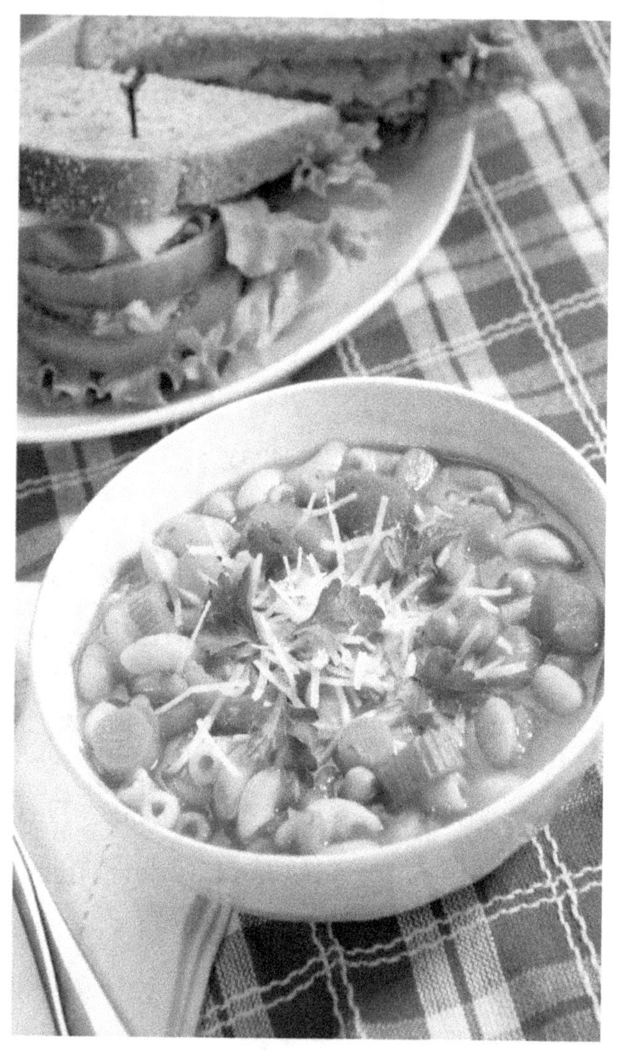

CHAPTER 7

BEVERAGES TO SOOTHE AND SIP

Peppermint Tea:

Ingredients:

- 1 peppermint tea bag or 1 tablespoon dried peppermint leaves
- 1 cup hot water

Instructions:

1. Place the peppermint tea bag or dried leaves in a cup.
2. Pour hot water over the tea bag or leaves.
3. Cover the cup and let it steep for about 5-10 minutes.
4. Remove the tea bag or strain the leaves.
5. Enjoy your soothing and digestive-friendly peppermint tea.

Chamomile Tea:

Ingredients:

- 1 chamomile tea bag or 1 tablespoon dried chamomile flowers
- 1 cup hot water

Instructions:

1. Place the chamomile tea bag or dried flowers in a cup.
2. Pour hot water over the tea bag or flowers.
3. Cover the cup and let it steep for about 5 minutes.
4. Remove the tea bag or strain the flowers.
5. Sip on the mild and calming chamomile tea.

Ginger Tea:

Ingredients:

- 1-inch piece of fresh ginger, thinly sliced (or 1 teaspoon dried ginger)
- 1 cup hot water
- Honey (optional, for sweetness)

Instructions:

1. Place the sliced ginger in a cup.
2. Pour hot water over the ginger.
3. Cover the cup and let it steep for about 5-10 minutes.
4. Remove the ginger slices.
5. Add honey if desired for sweetness.
6. Enjoy the warm and digestive-aiding ginger tea.

Ingredients:

- 1 fennel tea bag or 1 tablespoon crushed fennel seeds
- 1 cup hot water

Instructions:

1. Place the fennel tea bag or crushed seeds in a cup.
2. Pour hot water over the tea bag or seeds.
3. Cover the cup and let it steep for about 5-10 minutes.
4. Remove the tea bag or strain the seeds.
5. Sip on the aromatic and stomach-soothing fennel tea.

Aloe Vera Juice:

Ingredients:

- 1 fresh aloe vera leaf (make sure it's organic and free from chemicals)
- 1 cup cold water
- 1-2 tablespoons honey or lemon juice (optional, for flavor)

Instructions:

1. Prepare the Aloe Vera Leaf:

- Wash the aloe vera leaf thoroughly under running water to remove any dirt or residue.
- Use a sharp knife to carefully remove the thorny edges of the leaf.
- Cut the aloe vera leaf into smaller sections, making it easier to work with.

2. **Extract the Gel:**

- Lay each section of the aloe vera leaf flat on a cutting board.

- Slice off the top green layer, exposing the clear gel underneath.

- Use a spoon to carefully scoop out the gel and place it in a clean bowl. Be cautious not to include any of the yellowish latex layer, as it can have a laxative effect and may not be suitable for those with diverticulitis.

3. **Blend the Gel:**

- Place the aloe vera gel in a blender.

- Add 1 cup of cold water and blend until you have a smooth liquid.

- If you'd like to enhance the flavor, you can add 1-2 tablespoons of honey or lemon juice to the blender and blend again.

4. **Strain (Optional):** For a smoother texture, strain the aloe vera juice through a fine-mesh strainer or cheesecloth into a clean container.

5. **Serve and Store:**

- Pour the aloe vera juice into a glass and drink it immediately.

- Any leftover juice can be stored in the refrigerator for up to a few days.

Cucumber Water:

Ingredients:

- 1 cucumber, washed and thinly sliced (peeling is optional)

- 8 cups of water

- Ice cubes (optional)

- Fresh mint leaves or a slice of lemon (optional, for added flavor)

Instructions:

1. **Prepare the Cucumber:** Wash the cucumber thoroughly. You can choose to peel it or leave the skin on for added fiber and nutrients. Thinly slice the cucumber into rounds.

2. **Combine Ingredients:** In a large pitcher, add the cucumber slices. If you like, you can also add a few fresh mint leaves or a slice of lemon for extra flavor.

3. **Add Water:** Pour 8 cups of cold water into the pitcher with the cucumber. If you prefer your cucumber water extra cold, you can add ice cubes at this point.

4. **Stir and Chill:** Give the mixture a gentle stir to distribute the cucumber slices evenly. Cover the pitcher and place it in the refrigerator to chill for at least 1-2

hours. This allows the flavors of the cucumber to infuse into the water.

5. **Serve:** When ready to serve, pour the cucumber water into glasses, and you can add more ice cubes or garnish with extra mint leaves or lemon slices if desired.

6. **Enjoy:** Sip on the refreshing cucumber water throughout the day to stay hydrated and enjoy the subtle cucumber flavor.

Coconut Water:

Ingredients:

- Fresh coconut (one or more, depending on how much coconut water you want)
- A sharp knife
- A container or glass

Instructions:

1. **Select a Fresh Coconut:** Look for a fresh, green coconut with no visible cracks or damage. It should feel heavy when you pick it up, indicating that it's full of coconut water.

2. **Prepare the Coconut:**

- Use a sharp knife to carefully cut off the top of the coconut, creating a small hole. Be cautious not to cut too deep into the coconut to avoid puncturing the inner flesh.

- Hold the coconut over a container or glass, allowing the coconut water to drain into it. You may need to tilt the coconut to get all the water out.

3. **Strain (Optional):** If you want to remove any small particles or pieces of

coconut shell, you can strain the coconut water through a fine-mesh strainer or cheesecloth into another container or glass.

4. **Serve and Enjoy:** Once you've collected the coconut water, you can enjoy it immediately. It's best served chilled. You can also store any leftover coconut water in the refrigerator for a day or two.

Homemade Electrolyte Drink:

Ingredients:

- 2 cups of water (filtered or boiled and cooled)
- 1/2 cup of unsweetened coconut water (or plain water if you prefer)
- 1-2 tablespoons of honey or maple syrup (for sweetness)
- 1/4 teaspoon of salt (sodium)

- 1/4 teaspoon of baking soda (sodium and bicarbonate)
- 1/4 teaspoon of potassium chloride (optional, for potassium)
- Juice of 1/2 lemon or lime (for flavor)

Instructions:

1. **Prepare the Ingredients:** Make sure all your ingredients are clean and ready to use.

2. **Mix the Dry Ingredients:** In a clean container, mix the salt, baking soda, and potassium chloride (if using). These ingredients provide essential electrolytes: sodium, bicarbonate, and potassium.

3. **Add Liquid Ingredients:** In a separate pitcher or container, combine the water, coconut water (or additional plain water), honey or maple syrup, and the juice of

half a lemon or lime. These ingredients provide hydration, sweetness, and flavor.

4. **Combine and Stir:** Slowly pour the dry electrolyte mix into the liquid mixture while stirring continuously. This ensures that the electrolytes are evenly distributed.

5. **Taste and Adjust:** Taste the homemade electrolyte drink and adjust the sweetness or tartness to your liking by adding more honey, lemon juice, or water if necessary.

6. **Chill (Optional):** You can refrigerate the homemade electrolyte drink for a refreshing and cooling effect. However, you can also serve it immediately if needed.

7. **Serve:** Pour the electrolyte drink into a glass and enjoy it slowly. Sip on it

throughout the day as needed to stay hydrated and replenish electrolytes.

Carrot and Ginger Juice:

Ingredients:

- 4-5 medium-sized carrots, washed and peeled
- 1-inch piece of fresh ginger, peeled
- 1/2 lemon, peeled (optional, for added flavor)
- 1/2 to 1 cup of water (adjust for desired consistency)
- Honey or maple syrup (optional, for sweetness)

Instructions:

1. **Prepare the Ingredients:** Wash and peel the carrots, peel the ginger, and cut

them into smaller pieces to make them easier to juice.

2. **Juice the Carrots and Ginger:** Using a juicer, juice the carrots and ginger together. If you prefer a slightly tangy flavor, you can also juice the lemon and add it to the mixture.

3. **Adjust Consistency:** Depending on your preference, you can adjust the consistency of the juice by adding water. Start with 1/2 cup and add more if needed to achieve your desired thickness.

4. **Sweeten (Optional):** If you'd like to add a touch of sweetness, you can stir in honey or maple syrup to taste. Start with a small amount and adjust as needed.

5. **Serve and Enjoy:** Pour the carrot and ginger juice into a glass and enjoy it immediately. You can also add ice cubes for a refreshing twist.

6. **Store (Optional):** If you have leftover juice, you can store it in the refrigerator in an airtight container for a day or two. Shake or stir before serving.

Minty Lemon Water:

Ingredients:

- 1 lemon, washed and sliced
- 10-12 fresh mint leaves
- 4-6 cups of water (adjust to taste)
- Ice cubes (optional)
- Honey or maple syrup (optional, for sweetness)

Instructions:

1. **Prepare the Ingredients:** Wash the lemon thoroughly, and then slice it into thin rounds. Wash the fresh mint leaves.

2. **Combine Ingredients:** In a large pitcher, add the lemon slices and fresh mint leaves.

3. **Muddle (Optional):** If you want a stronger mint flavor, gently muddle the mint leaves with the back of a spoon or a muddler to release their aroma before adding the water.

4. **Add Water:** Pour the cold water into the pitcher with the lemon and mint. Adjust the amount of water to your taste preferences.

5. **Sweeten (Optional):** If you prefer a slightly sweet flavor, you can add honey or maple syrup to the pitcher. Start with a small amount, stir, and taste. Add more sweetener if needed.

6. **Stir:** Give the mixture a gentle stir to combine the ingredients.

7. **Chill (Optional):** You can refrigerate the pitcher for about an hour if you prefer your minty lemon water to be chilled.

8. **Serve:** Pour the minty lemon water into glasses filled with ice cubes (if desired) and garnish with an extra sprig of mint or a lemon slice.

9. **Enjoy:** Sip on the refreshing minty lemon water throughout the day to stay hydrated and enjoy its soothing flavor.

Decaffeinated Green Tea:

Ingredients:

- 1 decaffeinated green tea bag or 1 teaspoon of decaffeinated green tea leaves
- 1 cup of hot water
- Honey or lemon (optional, for flavor)

Instructions:

1. **Boil Water:** Bring a cup of water to a boil. Once the water reaches a rolling boil, remove it from the heat source.

2. **Add Tea:** Place the decaffeinated green tea bag or tea leaves into a cup.

3. **Pour Hot Water:** Pour the hot water over the tea bag or tea leaves in the cup.

4. **Steep:** Cover the cup with a lid or saucer and let the tea steep for about 3-5 minutes. Steeping time can vary depending on your taste preference; steeping for a shorter time will result in a milder flavor.

5. **Remove Tea Bag or Strain:** If you used a tea bag, remove it from the cup. If you used tea leaves, strain the tea into another cup to remove the leaves.

6. **Add Flavor (Optional):** If desired, you can add honey or a squeeze of lemon to your decaffeinated green tea for added flavor. Adjust the sweetness and tartness to your liking.

7. **Serve:** Your decaffeinated green tea is ready to enjoy. Drink it slowly and savor the soothing and mild flavor.

8. **Enjoy:** Sip on your decaffeinated green tea as needed throughout the day. It can be a calming and hydrating choice for those with diverticulitis.

Warm Broths:

Ingredients:

- 1 whole chicken (about 3-4 pounds), preferably organic
- 1 onion, peeled and halved
- 2 carrots, washed and cut into chunks
- 2 celery stalks, washed and cut into chunks
- 2 cloves garlic, peeled and smashed (optional)
- 1 bay leaf
- Fresh parsley (optional)
- Salt and pepper to taste
- Water

Instructions:

1. **Prepare the Chicken:**
- Rinse the chicken thoroughly under cold running water.
- Remove any giblets or excess fat from the chicken's cavity.

2. **Place Ingredients in a Large Pot:** In a large soup pot or stockpot, place the whole chicken, onion halves, carrots, celery, garlic (if using), bay leaf, and a few sprigs of fresh parsley (if available).

3. **Add Water:** Pour enough cold water into the pot to cover the chicken and vegetables by about 2 inches. This will depend on the size of your pot and chicken.

4. **Bring to a Simmer:** Place the pot over medium-high heat and bring the mixture to a gentle simmer.

5. **Skim Foam (Optional):** As the broth begins to simmer, you may notice some foam rising to the surface. Skim off this foam with a spoon and discard it.

6. **Simmer Gently:** Once the foam is removed, reduce the heat to low and let the broth simmer gently for about 1.5 to

2 hours. The longer it simmers, the richer the flavor will be.

7. **Season and Strain:**

- Season the broth with salt and pepper to taste, adding a little at a time and tasting as you go.

- Remove the chicken and vegetables from the broth using a slotted spoon or tongs. Discard the solids.

8. **Strain the Broth:** Strain the broth through a fine-mesh strainer or cheesecloth into a clean container or pot to remove any remaining impurities.

9. **Cool and Store:** Allow the broth to cool to room temperature. You can then refrigerate it in airtight containers or freeze it for later use.

Golden Milk:

Ingredients:

- 1 cup unsweetened almond milk (or a milk of your choice)
- 1/2 teaspoon ground turmeric
- 1/4 teaspoon ground cinnamon
- 1/8 teaspoon ground ginger
- A pinch of ground black pepper (optional)
- 1-2 teaspoons honey or maple syrup (optional, for sweetness)

Instructions:

1. **Combine Ingredients:** In a small saucepan, whisk together the unsweetened almond milk, ground turmeric, ground cinnamon, ground ginger, and a pinch of ground black pepper (if using). Black pepper can enhance the absorption of curcumin, the active compound in turmeric.

2. **Warm the Mixture:** Place the saucepan over low to medium heat. Warm the mixture while stirring continuously. Be careful not to let it boil; you just want it to be hot and steaming.

3. **Sweeten (Optional):** If you prefer your golden milk slightly sweetened, add honey or maple syrup to taste. Start with a small amount and adjust to your preference.

4. **Stir Well:** Continue to stir the golden milk until it's well blended and heated to your desired temperature.

5. **Serve:** Pour the golden milk into a mug and enjoy it while it's warm.

Rice Water:

Ingredients:

- 1/2 cup white rice (preferably long-grain)
- 4 cups water
- A pinch of salt (optional, for flavor)

Instructions:

1. **Rinse the Rice:** Place the white rice in a fine-mesh strainer and rinse it thoroughly under cold running water until the water runs clear. This helps remove excess starch.

2. **Boil the Rice:** In a medium-sized saucepan, add the rinsed rice and 4 cups of water. If you'd like, you can add a pinch of salt for flavor. Stir briefly.

3. **Simmer the Rice:** Place the saucepan over medium-high heat and bring the mixture to a boil. Once it boils, reduce the heat to low to maintain a gentle simmer.

4. **Cook the Rice:** Allow the rice to simmer for about 15-20 minutes or until the rice is fully cooked and the water becomes cloudy. Stir occasionally to prevent sticking.

5. **Strain the Rice Water:** Once the rice is fully cooked, remove it from the heat. Using a fine-mesh strainer or colander, strain the rice water into a clean container or bowl. Discard the cooked rice or save it for another use.

6. **Cool the Rice Water:** Allow the rice water to cool to a comfortable temperature before consuming it. You can place it in the refrigerator to chill it further if desired.

7. **Serve:** Pour the plain rice water into a glass and drink it slowly. You can enjoy it warm or cold, as you prefer.

Ingredients:

- 1/2 cup plain low-fat yogurt (ensure it's suitable for your dietary needs)
- 1/2 cup unsweetened almond milk (or a milk of your choice)
- 1 ripe banana, peeled and sliced
- 1/2 cup cooked and cooled oatmeal (avoid adding nuts or seeds if you have diverticulitis)
- 1/2 cup cooked and peeled apple (steamed or baked until soft)
- 1/2 teaspoon ground cinnamon (optional, for flavor)
- Honey or maple syrup (optional, for sweetness)
- Ice cubes (optional)

Instructions:

1. **Prepare the Ingredients:** Cook the oatmeal and apple in advance, allowing them to cool to room temperature before using. Make sure the banana is ripe and ready to be sliced.

2. **Combine Ingredients:** In a blender, add the plain yogurt, unsweetened almond milk, sliced banana, cooled oatmeal, cooked apple, and ground cinnamon (if using).

3. **Sweeten (Optional):** If you prefer your smoothie to be slightly sweetened, add honey or maple syrup to taste. Start with a small amount and adjust to your liking.

4. **Blend:** Blend all the ingredients until you have a smooth and creamy texture. If the smoothie is too thick, you can add a few ice cubes or more almond milk to reach your desired consistency.

5. **Taste and Adjust:** Taste the smoothie and adjust the sweetness or cinnamon flavor as needed.

6. **Serve:** Pour the smoothie into a glass and enjoy it immediately.

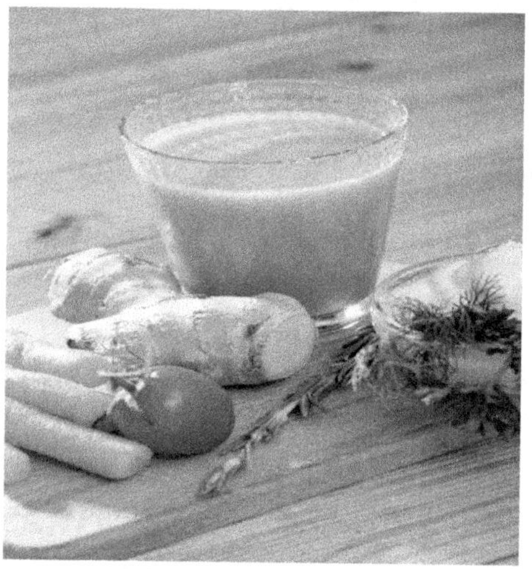

CHAPTER 8

MAINTAINING A DIVERTICULITIS DIET LONG-TERM

Tips for staying on track

Staying on track in recovery from diverticulitis involves making long-term dietary and lifestyle changes to reduce the risk of future flare-ups. Here are some tips to help you stay on track:

1. **Follow the Diverticulitis Diet:** Continue to follow the dietary recommendations provided by your healthcare professional or registered dietitian. This typically involves a high-fiber diet that includes plenty of fruits, vegetables, whole grains, and lean proteins while avoiding trigger foods.

2. **Stay Hydrated:** Drink plenty of water throughout the day. Proper hydration is essential for maintaining regular bowel movements and preventing constipation, which can exacerbate diverticulitis symptoms.

3. **Gradually Increase Fiber:** If you've been advised to increase your fiber intake, do so gradually. Rapidly adding a lot of fiber to your diet can cause bloating and discomfort. Add fiber-rich foods slowly over time.

4. **Portion Control:** Pay attention to portion sizes to avoid overeating. Smaller, more frequent meals can be easier on your digestive system than large, heavy meals.

5. **Chew Food Thoroughly:** Take your time to chew your food thoroughly. Proper chewing helps with digestion and

reduces the risk of irritation to the digestive tract.

6. **Limit Trigger Foods:** Continue to avoid foods that can trigger diverticulitis symptoms. Common trigger foods include nuts, seeds, popcorn, and spicy or fried foods. Always check with your healthcare provider about when and if it's safe to reintroduce these foods.

7. **Manage Stress:** Chronic stress can worsen digestive symptoms. Practice stress-reduction techniques such as deep breathing, meditation, yoga, or mindfulness to help manage stress.

8. **Regular Exercise:** Engage in regular physical activity, as exercise can promote healthy digestion and reduce the risk of constipation. Discuss appropriate exercise options with your healthcare provider.

9. **Medication Adherence:** If your healthcare provider has prescribed medications to manage diverticulitis or related conditions, be sure to take them as directed.

10. **Regular Check-Ups:** Attend regular follow-up appointments with your healthcare provider to monitor your condition and discuss any concerns or changes in your symptoms.

11. **Keep a Food Diary:** Consider keeping a food diary to track what you eat and any associated symptoms. This can help you identify specific trigger foods and make necessary adjustments to your diet.

12. **Stay Informed:** Stay informed about diverticulitis and digestive health. Knowledge can empower you to make informed decisions about your diet and lifestyle.

13. **Support System:** Seek support from friends, family, or support groups. It can be helpful to share your experiences and challenges with others who may have similar conditions.

14. **Be Patient:** Recovery from diverticulitis can take time, and there may be occasional setbacks. Be patient with yourself and stay committed to your health and well-being.

Tracking your progress

Tracking your progress in recovery from diverticulitis is essential to ensure that you're making positive strides and maintaining a healthy lifestyle. Here are some ways to track your progress:

1. **Symptom Journal:** Keep a daily or weekly journal to record your symptoms

and their severity. Note any changes or patterns in your symptoms over time. This can help you and your healthcare provider identify triggers or improvements.

2. **Dietary Record:** Maintain a food diary to track what you eat and drink. Note any foods that seem to worsen or improve your symptoms. This can be valuable information for making dietary adjustments.

3. **Bowel Movement Log:** Keep track of your bowel movements. Note the frequency, consistency, and any discomfort or pain associated with them. This can help assess your digestive health.

4. **Medication and Supplement Records:** If you're taking medications or supplements prescribed by your

healthcare provider, keep a record of when and how you take them. Note any side effects or changes in your symptoms.

5. **Weight and Measurements:** Regularly weigh yourself and track your measurements if desired. While weight isn't the sole indicator of progress, it can be a useful metric to monitor.

6. **Physical Activity Log:** Maintain a log of your physical activity. Track the type of exercise, duration, and intensity. This can help ensure you're staying active and monitor your fitness progress.

7. **Mood and Stress Levels:** Record your mood and stress levels regularly. Chronic stress can affect digestive health, so tracking your emotional well-being is important.

8. **Appointments and Tests:** Keep a calendar of healthcare appointments, including follow-up visits with your healthcare provider and any scheduled tests or procedures. This ensures you stay on top of your medical care.

9. **Sleep Patterns:** Track your sleep patterns, including the duration and quality of your sleep. Poor sleep can impact your overall well-being and digestion.

10. **Wellness Goals:** Set specific wellness goals related to your diverticulitis recovery. These could include dietary changes, exercise routines, stress reduction strategies, or weight management goals. Regularly assess your progress toward these goals.

11. **Consult with Your Healthcare Provider:** Share your progress tracking

with your healthcare provider during follow-up appointments. They can provide guidance and make adjustments to your treatment plan as needed.

12. **Celebrate Achievements:** Acknowledge and celebrate your achievements along the way. Whether it's reaching a dietary milestone, increasing your exercise intensity, or experiencing fewer symptoms, recognizing progress can be motivating.